Treating People with Anxiety and Stress

a practical guide for primary care

Greg Wilkinson

FRCP (Edin), FRCPsych

Professor of Liaison Psychiatry
University of Liverpool

Bruce Moore

MRCPsych

Research Specialist Registrar
Royal Liverpool University Hospital

and

Pascale Moore

DClinPsychol

Principal Clinical Neuropsychologist
The Walton Centre for Neurology and Neurosurgery
Liverpool

D1387416

RADCLIFFE MEDICAL PRESS

© 2000 Wilkinson, Moore and Moore

Radcliffe Medical Press
18 Marcham Road, Abingdon, Oxon OX14 1AA

British Library Cataloguing in Publication Data
A catalogue record for this book is available from the British Library.

ISBN 1 85775 139 6

Typeset by Joshua Associates Ltd, Oxford
Printed and bound by Biddles Ltd, Guildford and King's Lynn

Contents

Preface

This book is about the recognition and treatment of anxiety and stress related disorders, and as such concerns itself with what a previous generation of doctors called 'neuroses'. This word was coined by William Cullen (1710–90), an Edinburgh physician who was interested in the neurological basis of mental disorder. The following century saw advances in the neuropathology of 'nervous diseases' such as the aphasias (Wernicke and Broca), confabulation (Korsakoff) and dementia (Alzheimer) to mention but a few. Despite this progress, the influence of psychodynamic theory removed neurotic disorders from the domain of the brain to the milieu of the mind, thus divorcing nervous disease from neurology. Thus the very 'neurosis' which has been birthed by neurology became the bane of medicine and the hobby of analysts. This ideological shift was evident in early 20th century medicine: neurological disorders like Huntingdon's chorea and Parkinson's disease were now somewhat disparagingly viewed as 'neurotic'. Indeed, when the anatomical abnormalities responsible for such disorders were first described, there was surprise bordering on disbelief.

At the close of the 20th century there remains the vestige of this ideological divide between what is organic and psychological, but progress in neuroscience is fast closing the gap. Stress is no longer seen as a fashionable ailment of the over-indulgent developed world. Rather, it is the product of a mismatch between individual capacity and environmental demands, associated with a characteristic neuroendocrine imbalance which leads to the sequelae described in the text. Nevertheless, this 'environmental mismatch' does not affect everyone in the same way, and genetic research has identified a pattern of hereditary vulnerability to the spectrum of anxiety disorders. Increasingly, neuroscientists from backgrounds such as experimental psychology, neurophysiology and psychiatry are coming together in pursuit of a common goal – to understand the mechanisms of nervous disease. Thus it has been shown that cognitive therapy affects the cortical distribution of thought processes, thereby altering the cognitive 'brain map', whilst pharmacotherapy targets brain areas involved in subjective experience.

These exciting discoveries also serve to unify the clinical disciplines involved in patient care, as each is seen as contributing a valuable component to the healing process.

For those patients who suffer the torments of anxiety and stress, it is hoped that this book will provide redress from the long polarised climate of professional rivalry, and offer the combined approach to therapy that each individual deserves. It is to all sufferers of anxiety and stress related disorders that this book is therefore dedicated.

Greg Wilkinson
Bruce Moore
Pascale Moore
August 1999

Acknowledgements

As with the companion/sister volume *Treating People with Depression* this book would not have been possible without the combined efforts of several people. Once again, we are grateful to Ms Denise Hargreaves for typing the text, and also to Dr Sandy Stuart (General Practitioner), Dr Sam Vovnik (Psychiatrist) and Dr James Riley (Clinical Psychologist) for taking the time to read and comment upon the text. In addition, we would like to extend our thanks to Radcliffe Medical Press, and in particular Jamie Etherington, for keeping a judicious and timely eye on the project.

Prologue

It is perhaps a testament to the guidance and advice, help and support of the consultant psychiatrist, my GP, and the concerted efforts by me the patient that I am now able to see past events in perspective.

There is little doubt that I became a patient (initially troubled with sleep problems) because my unusually sad set of circumstances of bereavement, tragic death and role of carer stretched me to my emotional limits, each set of circumstances adding relentlessly and onerously to the next. In short, constraints of family responsibility have held me in an unavoidable state of tension for many years.

The explanation 'when pressure exceeds our ability to cope' seems most aptly to describe my state of stress and anxiety. Regarded as a seemingly strong person in both my personal and professional life, it was difficult to understand and accept that the negative emotions and physiological effects of excess pressure were causing health problems (and that it was now me who needed to be helped).

It is, of course, well documented that the prolonged role of carer eventually takes its toll on the carer's health, both physical and emotional. Perhaps not so well known is that it is all too easy for carers to forget to take remedial action to safeguard themselves when, day after day, they have unremitting emotional concerns for those for whom they are responsible.

I had not judged that I could be so susceptible to an unwanted state of anxiety and attendant symptoms of weight loss, poor sleep pattern, damaging personal relationships, impatience, digestive disturbances, and of course extreme tension.

To be in a downward spiral of negative emotions when all measures of self-help seem exhausted caused much misery, and there was apparently no way up. It has been at such times of emotional unhappiness with the feeling of precariously walking a tightrope between depression and stress-related anxiety that the added fear of a depressive illness has seemed only too real.

Perhaps most crucial to it all in my case is the emotional stress caused by the lack of intimate, confiding relationships – the very people lost to me through death and for whom I was grieving; and those for whom I was now caring were themselves trapped behind their own deteriorating condition and infirmity. So it was that I came to rely on professional help, opting for self-help remedial action rather than medication.

The definition that stress is the result of the difference between expectation and reality is my best practical and emotional yardstick. There is a tendency in many of us with busy lives and responsibilities to be unrealistically too optimistic in extending the expectations of what is possible beyond the time allowed. Constantly being on 'over-load' brings its own unwelcome consequences on health, and my experience is that mis-management of time with unrealistic goals can be a sure cause of panic and other unwanted symptoms.

With this in mind, of great importance now is the way forward, remembering to use measures of control to exclude anxiety from the equation.

Moreover, I firmly intend to resist the temptation to 'anticipate' every eventuality; and furthermore, to adopt a more passive approach of 'Let's wait and see what happens . . .', and allow events to unfold.

My eventual goal is to be optimistic enough to view new ventures and concepts as a challenge within, of course, realistic parameters!

Anonymous

1
Introduction

For some general practitioners (GPs) the concept of a psychiatric diagnosis is not one that makes much sense. This idea is encapsulated in the famous dictum attributed to Marshall Marinker:

> You are a case of diazepam – have some anxiety.

As an illustration of this, Raynes (1979) compared the contribution of presenting symptoms and the exploration of these by GPs, together with that of diagnosis, with the prescribing of psychotropic drugs. The focus of patient and GP on both physical and emotional issues was the most common characteristic of consultations leading to the prescription of a psychotropic drug. This focus occurred more frequently than either the diagnosis of a psychological disorder or the presentation of symptoms classed as psychosocial.

Also, data from the United States National Ambulatory Medical Care Survey show that the majority of psychotropic drugs and psycho-therapy/listening are provided in consultations during which no diagnosis of mental disorder is recorded.

Interobserver variation in assessment of mental ill health

In fact, there is a high degree of interobserver variation among GPs in the assessment of mental ill health. In Jenkins et al.'s (1988) study, using ICHPPC-2 (WONCA 1979), when experienced GPs viewed a videotape of a GP–patient consultation, 40% diagnosed neurotic depression, 25% 'anxiety depression', 10% syncope, faint or headache, 1% affective psychosis/hysterical or hypochondriacal disorder/other neurosis/ adjustment reaction and 20% made no diagnosis.

The differences between GPs and psychiatrists in their assessment of patients with neurotic disorders is illustrated by data from a study of the outcome of neurotic illness in general practice (*see* Table 1.1). Seventeen of the psychiatric 'cases' did not qualify as such (as recognised by a psychiatrist) despite the presence of psychiatric symptoms. These patients gave a history of improvement between identification by the GP and assessment by the psychiatrists.

Table 1.1 One hundred patients with neurotic disorders

General practitioner	Assessment	Psychiatrist
33	anxiety	33
38	depression	56
17	psychogenic	3
5	insomnia	2
	others	6

Adapted from Mann *et al.* (1981).

The differences between the GP and psychiatric diagnostic categories could be summarised as follows: psychiatrists diagnosed more people as suffering from depression than the GPs, finding such people from within the group classed as anxious by the GPs; and psychiatrists diagnosed anxiety states in many of the people classed as having physical disorders of psychogenic origin and insomnia by the GPs.

Improving detection of psychiatric illness in general practice

Goldberg and colleagues (quoted in Goldberg and Huxley, 1980) conducted a series of studies on the determinants of the ability of GPs to detect psychiatric illness, make accurate ratings of psychiatric symptoms and also the effects of training GPs to recognise psychiatric illness with increased accuracy (*see* Boxes 1.1 and 1.2).

A tendency to avoid or make many psychiatric diagnoses was due to factors other than those determining accuracy of diagnosis, i.e. physicians placing great emphasis on psychiatric questions make illness assessments more frequently but are not more accurate.

Box 1.1 Individual characteristics associated with detection of psychiatric morbidity

- Patients:
  - – Female
  - – Middle-aged
  - – Unemployed
  - – Separated, divorced, widowed
  - – Seen frequently before
  - – Severe disorders
- Doctors:
  - – Interest and concern
  - – Conservatism
- Family practice trainees:
  - – Self-confident and outgoing
  - – High academic ability
  - – Directive techniques
  - – Realistic concepts

Adapted from Goldberg *et al.* (1988).

Box 1.2 Interview style and accuracy of detection

- make eye contact
- clarify complaint
- direct questions for physical complaints
- open to closed questioning style
- empathic style
- sensitive to verbal and non-verbal cues
- avoid reading case notes
- deal with over-talkativeness
- do not concentrate on past history

Adapted from Goldberg *et al.* (1988).

Scales for detecting anxiety (and depression) in general practice

To aid GPs in better recognition of mental illness, short scales have been devised by Goldberg *et al.* (1988) as dimensional measures of the severity of anxiety and depression (*see* Boxes 1.3 and 1.4).

Box 1.3 Anxiety scale

- Have you felt keyed-up/on-edge?
- Have you been worrying a lot?
- Have you been irritable?
- Have you had difficulty relaxing?
- If yes to two of the above, go on to ask:
  - Have you been sleeping poorly?
  - Have you had headaches or neck aches?
  - Have you had any of the following: trembling, tingling, dizzy spells, sweating, frequency, diarrhoea?
  - Have you been worried about your health?
  - Have you had difficulty falling asleep?

Box 1.4 Depression scale

- Have you had low energy?
- Have you had loss of interest?
- Have you lost confidence in yourself?
- Have you felt hopeless?
- If yes to any question, go on to ask:
  - Have you had difficulty concentrating?
  - Have you lost weight (due to poor appetite)?
  - Have you been waking early?
  - Have you felt slowed up?
  - Have you tended to feel worse in the mornings?

Adapted from Goldberg *et al.* (1988).

There is a score of one for each positive response; anxiety and depression scores are added. Patients with anxiety scores of 5 or depression scores of 2 have a 50% chance of having a clinically important disorder. Above these scores the probability rises sharply.

Classifying anxiety in general practice

Analysis of longitudinal records of anxiety and depression diagnosed by GPs in the second National Morbidity Survey tends to confirm that there is wide disagreement among GPs.

Diagnostic difficulties seem to arise with particular force at the 'minor' end of the spectrum of psychiatric morbidity, particularly where the distinction between illness, distress and 'disgust with life in general' remains unresolved (Shepherd and Wilkinson, 1988).

If current classification schemes appear unsatisfactory, this is largely because most diagnostic systems have been developed from the study of hospital patients suffering from 'major' disorders. Thus prevailing classifications fail to do justice to the wide range of illness.

International classification of health problems in primary care

The tenth edition of the International Classification of Diseases for Primary Health Care (ICD-10 PHC) represents an evolving taxonomy of family medicine, and also provides guidelines for the care of mental disorders. Relevant sections from ICD-10 PHC are given in the appendix to each chapter, where applicable.

These criteria are intended to improve the accuracy and reliability of statistics from primary care medicine, but hard edges have been put to diagnostic concepts, many of which in reality have blurred borders. In addition, the definitions provided are not intended to serve as a guide to diagnosis; the primary purpose of the classification is to reduce chances of miscoding after a diagnosis has been made and not to eliminate the possibility of diagnostic error.

For additional comparison the appendix shows rather more detailed classifications from the fourth edition of the American Psychiatric Association's (1994) Diagnostic and Statistical Manual of Mental Disorders (DSM-IV), as well as the tenth edition of the World Health Organisation's International Classification of Diseases (ICD-10). These are mainly intended for use by psychiatrists working in psychiatric settings, but have become popular as a standard set of criteria, and are included to complement the International Classification of Health Problems for Primary Care (ICHPPC) classification and to present another approach, which although probably more reliable is certainly not necessarily more valid in a general practice context.

Training to improve psychiatric skills

Gask and colleagues (1987, 1988) have devised courses designed to improve the psychiatric interviewing skills of both established GPs and trainees. Participants were instructed in a problem-based consultation model using audiotape and videotape feedback of real consultations in a group setting.

Evaluation demonstrated significant improvements in GPs' and trainees' psychiatric interviewing skills after training. Trainees who were below average before training tended to show the greatest improvement.

The authors suggest that GP trainers could be trained to provide a similar teaching experience for their own trainees. Group video feedback training appeared to be as effective as one-to-one video feedback training in improving the psychiatric interviewing skills of GP trainees, and could be more widely employed in general practice vocational training.

Appendix 1A

Classification of anxiety disorders in ICD-10 (1992)

ICD-10 classifies anxiety disorders under 'other anxiety disorders' within the general rubric of 'Neurotic, stress-related and somatoform disorders'. These disorders are categorised as follows:

- **F40**   **Phobic anxiety**
  - F40.0   Agoraphobia
  - F40.1   Social phobia
  - F40.2   Specific phobias
  - F40.8/9 Other/unspecified phobic anxiety

- **F41**   **Other anxiety disorders**
  - F41.0   Panic disorder
  - F41.1   Generalised anxiety disorder (GAD)
  - F41.2   Mixed anxiety and depressive disorder
  - F41.3   Other mixed anxiety disorders
  - F41.8/9 Other/unspecified anxiety disorders

- **F42**   **Obsessive-compulsive disorder**
  - F42.0   Obsessive thoughts or ruminations
  - F42.1   Compulsive acts or rituals
  - F42.2   Mixed obsessional thoughts and acts
  - F42.8/9 Other/unspecified

- **F43**   **Reaction to severe stress and adjustment disorders**
  - F43.0   Acute stress reaction
  - F43.1   Post-traumatic stress disorder
  - F43.2   Adjustment disorders
  - F43.8/9 Other/unspecified.

Generalised Anxiety Disorder (GAD)

According to ICD-10 GAD is characterised by anxiety that is generalised and persistent, but not restricted to, or even predominating in, any particular environmental circumstances (i.e. it is 'free-floating'). The dominant symptoms are variable but include complaints of persistent nervousness, trembling, muscular tensions, sweating, light-headedness, palpitations, dizziness and epigastric discomfort. Fears that the patient or a relative will shortly become ill or have an accident are often expressed.

The research diagnostic criteria for GAD are defined as follows:

- There must have been a period of at least six months with prominent tension, worry and feelings of apprehension about everyday events and problems

- At least four of the symptoms listed below must be present, at least one of which must be from items 1–4:

  (1) **Autonomic arousal symptoms**
    - palpitations or pounding heart, or accelerated heart rate
    - sweating
    - trembling or shaking
    - dry mouth (not due to medication or dehydration)

  (2) **Symptoms involving chest and abdomen**
    - difficulty breathing
    - feeling of choking
    - chest pain or discomfort
    - nausea or abdominal distress

  (3) **Symptoms involving mental state**
    - feeling dizzy, unsteady, faint or light-headed
    - feeling that objects are unreal (derealisation) or that the self is distant (depersonalisation)
    - fear of losing control, 'going crazy' or passing out
    - fear of dying

  (4) **General symptoms**
    - hot flushes or cold chills
    - numbness or tingling sensations
    - muscle tension or aches and pains
    - restlessness and inability to relax
    - feeling on edge
    - a sensation of a lump in the throat

  (5) **Other non-specific symptoms**
    - exaggerated startle response
    - difficulty in concentrating due to worrying or anxiety
    - persistent irritability
    - difficulty in geting to sleep due to worrying

- The disorder does not meet the criteria for panic disorder, phobic anxiety, obsessive-compulsive or hypochondriacal disorder

- The disorder is not due to a physical illness such as hyperthyroidism, organic mental disorder or substance use.

Appendix IB

Classification of anxiety disorders in DSM-IV (1994)

DSM-IV, in contrast to ICD-10, classifies anxiety under the more specific rubric of 'anxiety disorders', which includes the following:

- panic disorder without agoraphobia
- panic disorder with agoraphobia
- agoraphobia without history of panic disorder
- specific phobia
- social phobia
- obsessive-compulsive disorder
- post-traumatic stress disorder
- acute stress disorder
- generalised anxiety disorder
- anxiety due to a general medical condition
- substance-induced anxiety disorder
- anxiety disorder not otherwise specified.

The diagnostic criteria for **Generalised Anxiety Disorder 300.02** are as follows:

- Excessive anxiety and worry (apprehensive expectation), occurring more days than not for at least six months, about a number of events or activities
- The person finds it difficult to control the worry
- The anxiety and worry are associated with at least three of the following six symptoms present for more days than not over the past six months
  - restlessness or being on edge
  - being easily fatigued

- difficulty concentrating or mind going blank
- irritability
- muscle tension
- sleep disturbance (particularly of onset)

- The focus of the anxiety and worry is not confined to specific situations

- The anxiety symptoms cause clinically significant distress or impairment in social, occupational or other important areas of functioning

- The disorder is not due to substance use or medical condition, and is not confined to co-occurrence with another mental disorder.

2
Assessment of anxiety disorders

Anxiety is a normal response to threat or stress. Such anxiety will usually improve performance and is colloquially referred to as being 'psyched-up'. Attempts to reduce this type of anxiety are likely to impair performance. Hence, an appropriate amount of arousal improves performance but an excess of anxiety impairs performance; this relationship between performance and arousal is summarised by the 'Yerkes–Dodson' law, which is characteristically represented as a graph, as shown in Figure 2.1.

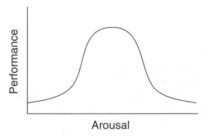

Figure 2.1 The 'Yerkes–Dodson' law, showing the relationship between performance and arousal.

Anxiety trait

This refers to the habitual tendency of an individual to be anxious and to worry. It describes a life-long personality trait and should be distinguished from the term 'state anxiety' which, if severe enough, usually signifies an illness.

Clinical anxiety

Often anxiety becomes too severe in degree, arrives unprovoked, or occurs repeatedly in specific yet innocuous situations. Such maladaptive patterns of anxiety are usually also associated with depression and together these symptoms constitute the most common psychiatric disorders in general practice.

Clinical anxiety:

- differs from normal anxiety partly by being more severe, but also because it occurs in the absence of obvious threat

- is a combination of psychological and physical disturbances which are severe and all-pervasive

- occurs either in attacks or as a persisting state.

Epidemiology of anxiety

The Epidemiological Catchment Area Study in the United States estimated the frequency of anxiety disorders at 8.3% of the general population, compared with the prevalence of depression which was diagnosed in 6% of the general population. At the same time, only 23% of those with anxiety and 18% of those with affective disorders were receiving treatment. This study underlines the high prevalence of untreated anxiety and depressive disorders. In general, women are more likely to suffer from anxiety disorders than men. The onset is often in early adult life although it may occur for the first time from childhood to old age. Anxiety states rarely develop for the first time after 40 years of age.

About 25% of patients seen in general practice have anxiety as a clinically significant component of their condition. About 5% of a practice population have phobias, of whom only a minority seek help. Similarly, about 3% of a general practice population have panic attacks.

Aetiology of anxiety

Neurobiology

Anxiety has generally been associated with the central noradrenergic system, in particular the locus coeruleus, which contains approximately 50–70% of the brain's noradrenaline-containing bodies. The locus coeruleus lies in the rostral pons adjacent to the cerebral aqueduct, and sends major efferent pathways to limbic areas, notably the amygdala and peri-hippocampal structures. It is also richly innervated by an inhibitory input of gamma-aminobutyric acid (GABA) neurones. Animal studies have shown that stimulating the rostral peri-aqueductal grey (PAG) produces a 'fight' response and stimulating the caudal PAG (the site of the locus coeruleus) produces a 'flight' response.

Neuro-anatomical and neurophysiological observations have lead to the idea that anxiety is mediated primarily via the noradrenergic system. It is suggested that antidepressants with significant inhibitory effects on the noradrenaline pathway may decrease anxiety by dampening noradrenergic hyper-responsiveness. This hypothesis is also consistent with benzodiazepine enhancement of inhibitory GABA input to the locus coeruleus. Positron emission tomography (PET) studies show that the major projections of the locus coeruleus are hypermetabolic when anxiety symptoms are intense. However, further studies are required to clarify the role of noradrenaline and serotonin in combination with many other neuroregulatory systems in the genesis of anxiety.

Main symptoms of anxiety

The main symptoms of anxiety are listed in Table 2.1.

Psychological features

Patients may complain of a variety of the following features of anxiety:

- apprehensiveness, fearing some unspecified disaster
- feeling tense, keyed-up or on-edge, ill-at-ease with a sense that something terrible is about to happen

Box 2.1 Other aetiological factors

Genetic	41% of monozygous twins had an anxiety disorder compared with only 4% of dizygous twins.
Personality	Some personalities are prone to anxiety and neuroticism.
Stressful event	Anxiety disorders often seem to begin in relation to stressful events and appear to become chronic when social problems persist.
Conditioning theory	Anxiety disorders may arise when fear responses become attached to previously neutral stimuli.
Cognitive theories	Anxiety disorders persist because of the way patients think about their symptoms; fears about symptoms lead to further anxiety and a vicious circle ensues.

Table 2.1

Psychological	Somatic
Anxiety	Tremor
Dread	Sweating
Apprehension	Palpitations
Fears	Dizziness
Excessive worry	Increased frequency of micturition
Insomnia	Increased frequency of bowel motions
Irritability	Hyperventilation
Obsessions	Muscular skeletal pain
Compulsions	Dry mouth
Depersonalisation	Muscle tension
Derealisation	Restlessness
Phobias	Tremulousness
Ruminations	Syncope
Panic	Chest pain
Impatience	Tightness in the chest
	Shortness of breath
	Paraesthesia
	Headache
	Vertigo

- worrying excessively, often about physical health – cancer and heart disease
- fearful about specific issues and situations, such as impending death of the individual or someone close
- easily startled and hypersensitive to noise
- irritable with family and friends, losing temper easily and being 'snappy'
- feeling restless, needing to be on the move
- unable to concentrate, wavering attention and forgetfulness, mind going 'blank'
- feeling helpless and unable to cope
- feeling panicky
- convinced they are going mad or about to lose their mind or lose control of their mental functioning.

Somatic features

These derive mainly from unwanted activity in the musculature, the limbic system and the autonomic (mainly sympathetic) nervous system, and are sometimes accompanied by metabolic changes.
    Patients may complain of:

- palpitations, throbbing pains in the chest and feelings of distension around the heart
- hot flushes or chills
- muscular tension
- a sensation of an inability to relax, together with motor restlessness
- initial insomnia, broken sleep with vivid dreams and nightmares
- tremor
- unreal feelings (depersonalisation and derealisation, in which patients complain of feeling strange, detached and alienated from their sense of identity or surroundings)
- 'globus hystericus' (a feeling of tightness or swelling in the throat)

- blushing
- pains and aches – often due to oesophageal gastric or musculoskeletal dysfunction
- cold, clammy hands and fingers
- dry mouth
- nausea
- diarrhoea, increased bowel activity, including the sensation of 'butterflies in the stomach'
- minor loss of appetite
- frequency or urgency of micturition
- impotence or frigidity
- shortness of breath, sense of suffocation or choking (this may lead to over-breathing which in turn may produce metabolic consequences such as faintness, muscle cramps, paraesthesia, tetany, etc)
- problems with sexual performance
- dizziness or light-headedness.

Anxiety and depression

Anxiety and depression are in most cases indistinguishable at the level of general practice and frequently precede or succeed each other in any given patient.

Symptoms more typical of depressive disorders are:

- lowered mood
- loss of interest
- thoughts of guilt and worthlessness
- loss of energy
- fatigue
- early morning wakening
- broken sleep

- indecision
- inability to concentrate
- somatic symptoms
- loss of appetite
- loss of libido
- suicidal ideas.

The main features which may help to discriminate between anxiety and depressive disorders are:

- previous episodes of either anxiety or depression
- absence or presence of diurnal variation in mood.

Differential diagnosis of anxiety

A number of psychiatric and physical disorders should be considered in the differential diagnosis of anxiety and the main differential diagnoses are shown in Boxes 2.2 and 2.3. Clearly, a variety of physical and psychosocial investigations may be required in order to help clarify what may at first be a confusing presenting clinical picture.

Depressive neurosis

Neurotic depression is characterised by disproportionate depression which has usually resulted from a distressing experience. There is often a preoccupation with a psychic trauma, which preceded the illness, e.g. loss of a cherished person or possession. Anxiety is also frequently present and mixed states of anxiety and depression are often included under this diagnostic category. This probably presents the most common clinical occurrence of anxiety.

- Associated depression is common.
- Drug misuse may also occur as a result of well-meaning but unnecessary over-prescription of medication, and abuse of alcohol and over-the-counter medication used for symptomatic relief.

Box 2.2 Psychiatric disorders

- depression
- schizophrenia
- pre-senile or senile dementia
- drug and alcohol dependence
- benzodiazepine dependence
- acute or chronic organic brain disorder
- alcohol withdrawal state
- alcoholic hallucinosis
- solvent abuse

Box 2.3 Physical disorders

- Endocrine
  - Thyrotoxicosis
  - Hypoglycaemia
  - Phaeochronocytoma
  - Carcinoid syndrome
  - Idiopathic hypoglycaemia
  - Insulinoma
- Cardiovascular
  - Angina
  - Myocardinal infarction
  - Mitral valve prolapse
  - Paroxysmal supraventricular tachycardia
  - Cardiac dysrhythmias
- Respiratory
  - Acute respiratory distress
  - Pulmonary embolism
  - Asthma
- Neurological
  - Acute brain syndrome
  - Cerebrovascular accident
  - Epilepsy, e.g. temporal lobe
- Medication related
  - Levadopa
  - Corticosteroids
  - Thyroxine
  - Bronchodilators
  - Caffeneism
  - Ephedrine
  - Amphetamine

- General decision-making and judgement are usually not impaired.

- Suicide is rarer in patients with anxiety than in those with depression.

Complications of anxiety

Dependence upon drugs, alcohol, tobacco, carers and services is found in the long-term for those with severe anxiety. The 10% who have dependence on alcohol and drugs have a worse outcome than the others. Such patients make frequent attendance at surgery with multiple complaints and receive a variety of symptomatic treatments. They are also often referred to a number of different hospital specialists. Moreover, there is an increased mortality in people with anxiety disorders. As well as suicide and accidents, there is a significantly increased mortality from natural causes. The most significant of these are from hypertension, peripheral vascular disease and coronary artery disease.

Long-term outcome of anxiety

There are very few studies on the long-term outcome of anxiety in a general practice setting, but in one such study of 100 chronic psychiatric patients identified in general practice, 34 patients were thought to have exhibited symptoms continuously or with frequent recurrence for at least 10 years (Cooper, 1965).

More recent studies of anxiety disorders seen in specialist settings indicate that certain factors are associated with poor outcome in terms of chronicity and relapse. Such factors are summarised below:

- concurrent personality disorder

- poor quality of relationships

- duration of illness

- concurrent depressive illness.

Children and anxiety

Children are not immune from stress and anxiety, or indeed from other psychiatric disorders. A previous generation of caring professionals tended to assume that children are more resilient to stressful situations than adults, somehow having an innate ability to 'bounce back' to normal, an assumption based largely on the erroneous collection of data from adults rather than from children themselves. Recent work, however, has demonstrated that children may be as likely to suffer from the same range of symptoms as adults when exposed to stressful and traumatic experiences, but young children may not have the necessary communication skills to express their feelings and symptoms adequately. Unfortunately, the present volume does not permit sufficient space to provide a detailed discussion of anxiety and stress in children, but the main areas of concern are outlined briefly below.

Assessment

Children tend to be more likely than adults to present with somatic complaints in response to stressful situations. This may reflect an element of conditioning (e.g. the early experience that it is more acceptable to be 'off school' on account of physical illness, as opposed to worries about being lonely, teased or bullied at school). A tendency to somatise may also reflect a degree of emotional immaturity, marked by an inability to interpret or read one's own internal feelings or mood; this is termed 'alexithymia' (literally, 'inability to read mood') and clearly this may persist into adulthood. Alexithymia has become an important concept in understanding a variety of somatising complaints, including conversion disorders and hypochondriasis.

Anxious children may therefore present with a variety of physical complaints, such as 'tummy pain', enuresis and exacerbations of atopic disorders (asthma and eczema), as well as behavioural problems such as hair pulling (trichotillomania), hair eating (which may lead to trichobezoar, or 'hair ball'), tics and conduct problems. Of course, it cannot be assumed that such presentations invariably represent under-lying anxiety, and it is always necessary for the clinician to be satisfied that physical illness is not present. It is because of the need to exclude physical illness that many younger schoolchildren receive a variety of physical investigations before it is concluded that they are suffering from anxiety.

Hence there is a fine balance to achieve in assessing children with non-specific symptoms; on the one hand, it is imperative not to miss a physical disorder, but on the other hand, it is also important to have an early awareness of non-organic dysfunction so that undue investigations may be avoided, as over-exposure to treatment settings may sow the seeds of subsequent abnormal illness behaviour. To illustrate these points, a sample case summary is given in Box 2.4.

The role of the family doctor

The GP is in many ways ideally placed to manage children with anxiety disorders, given the unique perspective on families which GPs have. Work with children constitutes about 25% of the workload in general practice. An average practice may look after at least 500 children, giving rise to about 1500 child consultations each year, with children under the age of five seeing their family doctor up to eight times per year on average. It has been pointed out that as over 90% of GPs provide antenatal care and 90% of children and mothers are registered with a GP, the family doctor has a crucial role to play in child care and can intervene at an early stage in the development of problems (Jezzard, 1995). It is in the area of early intervention that family doctors probably have the greatest impact in the lives not only of children, but of all of their patients. Some of the advantages of general practice in relation to child mental health problems are summarised in Box 2.5.

Children in the surgery

It is clear that GPs have a unique role to play in managing childhood disorders, and in the case of anxiety and other emotional and behavioural difficulties, the family doctor is best placed to provide early intervention. However, as mentioned previously, children may present in a variety of ways other than saying 'Doctor, I'm stressed!'. Moreover, children may present differently at varying ages and levels of maturity, a fact that places considerable demands on the judgement and perspicacity of even the most experienced doctors. To help provide a framework for assessing children, Markus et al. (1991) have compiled a useful summary of common emotional and behavioural problems that may present to GPs, as shown in Box 2.6.

GP intervention

The most crucial aspect of managing anxiety and stress-related disorders is to try and understand the social and family context in which the patient presents, a function which many GPs are well placed to perform.

Box 2.4 Case study of childhood anxiety presenting with a somatic complaint

Matthew was 9 years old and had already spent several weeks as an in-patient on the children's ward at a major teaching hospital. He had missed almost an entire term from school whilst undergoing various investigations for abdominal pain, which had begun 6 months previously. Following appendicectomy, histopathology had revealed a normal appendix and all other investigations, including biopsy of the intestinal mucosa, were normal. The ward was generally bright and cheerful, with plenty of things to occupy the children, including 3 hours per day of education time. There was unrestricted visiting and the staff, who formed a highly motivated team, made every effort to enhance the quality of life of their young patients. However, in Matthew's case it was noticed that whenever he was approached by a member of the medical or nursing staff, whether to offer pain relief or just to talk generally, he would suddenly alter his disposition from one of animated interest to one of misery. Moreover, staff noticed that after visiting time Matthew would often be seen alone and crying quietly in a corner, although he was never able to say why. In view of these findings, it was decided to refer the case to the child mental health team, and a comprehensive psychological assessment was made, involving Matthew's family.

In light of this assessment, it was discovered that the abdominal pain had arisen around the time that Matthew's father had left home a little over 6 months ago. His father frequently promised to return home to see Matthew, but never did, and when Matthew was admitted to hospital he apparently promised to visit him, but again never did. It was understood that the original 'tummy pain' was a psychosomatic response to an abrupt loss of his father, and that subsequent episodes, both of pain and crying, were related to repeated times when the boy was let down by his father. When it was explained to Matthew that his body, as well as his mind, was terribly upset at not seeing his father, he was finally able to express his feelings of utter frustration and sobbed for several minutes before he was reassured that he would be able to get better at home. Unfortunately the father did not engage either in the assessment or follow-up, but Matthew and his mother were given four sessions of direct contact with the child psychologist over the next few weeks and he was able to resume school the following term, with no subsequent episodes of severe abdominal pain.

> **Box 2.5** Advantages of general practice in relation to child mental health problems
>
> • GPs have an intergenerational perspective
> • GPs have regular opportunities to observe child–parent relationships
> • general practice is seen as less stigmatising
> • contact levels present many opportunities for early intervention
> • two-thirds of all family planning is received in general practice
> • GPs meet the male partner in four out of five family units
> • over 40% of patients have been looked after by the same GP for over 20 years
> • children under the age of five are seen by their GP up to eight times per year
> • babies are seen every 6–7 weeks on average
> • families are seen interacting at stressful times
>
> Adapted from Jezzard (1995).

However, a GP's contact time with each patient is limited and thus may not allow for a full assessment of the child's situation in relation to family, school and peer groups. For this reason many GPs, particularly in the fundholding practices of the early and mid-1990s, have developed child and family counselling services within the primary care setting; such initiatives have immediate cost advantages, but have been criticised for placing an inappropriate burden on the skills of counsellors who may not always be equipped or trained to deal with the more complex cases (Sibbald *et al.*, 1993).

Nevertheless, the large majority of cases of childhood anxiety are remediable in the primary care context, and need not be referred for specialist child mental health care. Very often it is sufficient to identify and communicate that stressors are underlying the problem; where this is communicated in an empathic way that confers respect for the genuine feelings and symptoms of the child, then usually the patient and family can be reassured that there is no physical illness. The events causing the anxiety may not be subject to change (as, for example, in the case history given on p. 22, of the 9–year-old boy with abdominal pain, whose father had left home), in which case simply gaining some insight into the origin of the problem can pave the way for a process of

---

Box 2.6 Common emotional and behavioural problems that may present to GPs

- Early childhood
  - Sleepless nights and nightmares
  - Temper tantrums and breath-holding
  - Clinging behaviour
  - Feeding and voiding problems
  - Bedwetting and soiling
- Middle childhood
  - School non-attendance
  - School underperformance (in the absence of low IQ)
  - Disobedience and aggressive behaviour
  - Social withdrawal and shyness
  - Recurrent abdominal pain and headaches
- Adolescence
  - School non-attendance
  - Delinquency
  - Substance abuse
  - Moodiness and irritability
  - Suicidal thoughts
  - Social anxieties and withdrawal
  - Eating problems

Adapted from Markus *et al.* (1991).

---

adaptation to the new situation. In other cases, the stressor may be changed, e.g. by addressing issues of bullying at school or relationship difficulties within the home. However, a proportion of more severe and chronic cases may be associated with an intense and disturbing traumatic experience (e.g. childhood sexual abuse) and clearly where such trauma is suspected, the clinician has a paramount duty of care to the child; in such cases it is always advisable to refer for specialist help and to inform the social services child protection team if abuse is suspected.

3
Treating generalised anxiety

The vast majority of anxiety disorders can, and should, be treated in general practice, either by the GP and the primary healthcare team (e.g. counsellor, physiotherapist, health visitor or practice nurse) or with help from the secondary mental health services (psychiatrist, community psychiatric nurse, social worker, clinical psychologist), preferably working within the general practice base.

The aim of treatment remains to relieve symptoms, help solve problems and improve social functioning in cost-effective ways. The first priority is to reduce and control the symptoms of anxiety. Thereafter it is necessary to introduce a treatment plan composed of further consultations, a mix of psychosocial and psychopharmacological treatment and some indicators of outcome so that longer term treatment can be instituted systematically if indicated.

Mental health professionals in the primary healthcare team

GPs are turning increasingly to nurses, social workers, clinical psychologists and counsellors rather than to psychiatrists for help for their patients with anxiety, depression and related problems (Wilkinson, 1988).

Nurses

GPs are the largest group referring patients to community psychiatric nurses. Community psychiatric nurses working in health centres are most commonly asked to help with patients with mood disorder. Two randomised, controlled trials have shown clinical and economic benefits of nurses treating patients with neuroses in the community. In one study community psychiatric nursing was compared with routine psychiatric out-patient follow-up over 18 months. Community psychiatric nursing resulted in an appreciable reduction in out-patient contact with psychiatrists and other staff, more discharges and a small increase in contacting GPs for prescribing. In the other study neurotic patients (mainly those with phobias and obsessive-compulsive disorders) had a better outcome 1 year after receiving behavioural psychotherapy from a nurse therapist than after routine treatment from a GP.

Practice nurses already provide much emotional support to patients with psychiatric and physical illness, although this is largely unrecorded. In addition health visitors are important in identifying and treating emotional problems in women who have recently given birth and in the elderly.

Social workers

Social work has been shown to be effective in the treatment of psychiatric disorders in general practice in two randomised, controlled trials. In one study, women suffering from acute or acute-on-chronic depression were referred either to a social worker attached to a general practice or for routine treatment by their GPs. Women with acute-on-chronic depression and marital difficulties benefited from treatment by social workers. In the other study, depressed patients in general practice were allocated to individual cognitive therapy, group cognitive therapy or a waiting list control group. Those who received cognitive therapy from a social worker did significantly better during the first year than those on the waiting list, but there was no significant difference between patients treated with group or individual cognitive therapy.

Clinical psychologists

GPs refer to clinical psychologists patients with difficulties ranging from anxiety to habit disorders. Patients showed high satisfaction with behavioural treatment and had a third to a half fewer consultations for advice or prescriptions for psychotropic drugs in the year after psychological intervention. Such benefits have been confirmed after 1 year of a randomised, controlled clinical and economic evaluation of a behaviourally oriented clinical psychology service in a health centre. Contact with a psychologist may have effects on referred patients and their families over the longer term, with decreases at 3 years in the number of prescriptions for psychotropic drugs for their children. Advantages have also been shown for specific psychological treatments in patients with depression and anxiety. Two controlled clinical trials have produced favourable early results for psychologists using cognitive therapy combined with antidepressants in treating depressive disorders. Group psychological treatment for anxiety has been compared with individual treatment; individual treatment was more effective in reducing anxiety, whereas service demands were considerably reduced by group treatment.

Counsellors

Growing numbers of counsellors are being recruited into primary care. Individual, family, group and marital counselling are used, and the counsellor's main aim is to offer the patient support and insight. Patients are also given the chance to learn new skills, such as relaxation, and vocational and educational guidance may be given. Several clinical accounts have shown the impact of counselling in general practice, e.g. on the subjective feelings of patients and GPs, and on reductions in the number of consultations and prescriptions for psychotropic drugs.

People with marital difficulties are more likely to contact a GP for help than any other social service, and several attachments of marriage guidance counsellors to general practice have been set up to encourage doctors to refer patients directly. These attachments seem to work well but the experience is limited to self-selected and atypical practices.

Benefits of mental health professionals in general practice

GPs are currently collaborating with paramedical workers, and statutory and voluntary agencies to provide the overwhelming bulk of psychiatric care in Britain. At the same time, GPs in many parts of Britain have no alternative to referring patients to a psychiatrist. While the evidence supports the effectiveness of the different therapeutic approaches, none of the studies is entirely satisfactory. Furthermore, cooperation and coordination between primary care and specialist mental health professionals is still underdeveloped and the cost-effectiveness of such collaborations remains largely unknown.

In a statistical meta-analysis of 11 British studies of specialist mental health treatment in general practice, the main finding was that treatment by specialist mental health professionals was about 10% more successful than that usually given by the GP (Balestrieri *et al.*, 1988). Counselling (including social work), behaviour therapy and general psychiatry proved to be similar in their overall effect. The influence of counselling seemed to be greatest on social functioning, whereas behaviour therapy seemed mainly to reduce contacts with the psychiatric out-patient services.

Family and friends

When possible and appropriate, specialised psychosocial help (e.g. mental health education, anxiety management) can best be provided at the patient's home where family or friends can be mobilised to enhance the likelihood of treatment adherence and success.

Patients who 'somatise' psychiatric distress

Patients often present to GPs with somatic symptoms for which no adequate physical cause can be found, and which are accompanied by the symptoms of an anxiety state or a depressive illness. These illnesses pose a major problem, but little is known about their management.

Goldberg *et al.* (1989) proposed a three-stage model to encourage patients to reattribute these symptoms and relate them to psychosocial problems. These stages are feeling understood, changing the agenda and making the link.

- **Feeling understood** derives from a full assessment, including exploration of social and family factors, health beliefs and a physical examination.

- **Changing the agenda** results from feedback of the assessment and physical symptoms and reframing the patient's complaints in the light of the symptoms and 'life-events'.

- **Making the link** is accomplished by making the connection between physical and emotional symptoms, explicit by explanation of the common physiological mechanisms, demonstrating the relationship between presenting symptoms, 'life-events' and 'here and now', and finally by 'projection' – if another family member has similar symptoms, it may be possible to get the patient to see that they have identified with the sick person.

Pharmacological treatment of anxiety

Beginning with the pharmacological approach to the treatment of anxiety does not reflect the importance of drugs compared with non-drug treatment. As mentioned previously, a large proportion of anxiety symptoms occurs in the context of everyday stressors and may respond to simple adjustments in the lifestyle of individuals; other more enduring cases benefit from talking treatments and adaptation to stressors. However, there remains a significant proportion of patients for whom non-drug approaches are insufficient.

Hence, drug treatment should be reserved for more severely ill patients, in whom symptoms are seriously interfering with social and occupational functioning, or who do not improve with other measures and continue to have unacceptable symptoms of anxiety. There is also evidence that combining drug treatment with talking therapy provides optimal outcome at long-term follow-up, with less chance of relapse.

Short-term treatment: benzodiazepines

These drugs should seldom be prescribed for more than 2–4 weeks because of the risk of dependence when given for long periods. With benzodiazepines up to 1 in 5 become long-term users. True dependence occurs in about one-third of these users, making the initial risk for dependence around 1 in 10. Several studies have suggested that benzodiazepines are no more effective than simple counselling, psychotherapy or anxiety management in over half of those people with anxiety who are normally considered to be suitable for anxiolytic drugs. The remainder probably need psychotropic drugs as well as non-drug treatments. In the most severe cases of GAD a long-acting benzodiazepine such as diazepam may be appropriate in doses ranging from 2 to 10 mg two or three times daily. Intermittent or prn (as required) doses may be appropriate. The likelihood of response can be assessed at 7 days and the drug stopped if there is no improvement. Even in short-term use the dose should be reduced and tapered-off to minimise rebound effects. The main points of benzodiazepine prescribing are summarised in Box 3.1.

Box 3.1   Benzodiazepines in GAD

Prescribing tips

- short-term use in severe anxiety; 2–4 weeks
- dose depending on severity; **Diazepam** 2–5 mg TDS (max. 10 mg TDS)
- institute psychological therapy or counselling
- tapered withdrawal depending on dosage and duration of use
- consider long-term selective serotonin reuptake inhibitor (SSRI) treatment (e.g. paroxetine)

Side-effects of benzodiazepines

Despite the undoubted efficacy of benzodiazepines in relieving anxiety symptoms, their use is complicated by marked adverse effects. During treament they may produce unwanted sedation as well as cognitive impairment and ataxia. Treatment withdrawal, even when tapered slowly, can lead to rebound anxiety symptoms, which all too often occasion restarting of treatment and can lead to dependence. Withdrawal effects and dependence are more likely to occur with high-potency benzodiazepines such as Lorazepam. The side-effects of benzodiazepines are shown in Box 3.2.

Box 3.2   Side-effects of benzodiazepines

- Common
  - ataxia
  - drowsiness
  - impaired concentration and memory
  - paradoxical disinhibition (e.g. aggression)
  - rebound anxiety on withdrawal
  - dependence
- Rare
  - headache
  - vertigo
  - gastrointestinal symptoms
  - jaundice
  - rash
  - visual disturbance
  - urinary retention.

Long-term treatment: 'antidepressants'

Many antidepressants are effective in controlling symptoms of anxiety, and in fact many were developed as anxiolytics but subsequently marketed as antidepressants in order to avoid prevalent negative attitudes towards 'sedatives'. Antidepressants which are most useful in treating anxiety tend to be those with marked serotonergic activity, of the older tricyclics clomipramine and imipramine are the best examples, most of the modern SSRIs are effective in the long-term treatment of anxiety, particularly those with a shorter half-life such as paroxetine. Such drugs may be effective in treating anxiety even in the absence of prominent depressive symtoms. These drugs should be considered in established cases of anxiety associated with significant impairment to social, work and domestic functioning.

In prescribing such long-term medication it is important to remember that onset of action is delayed and that SSRIs may cause some insomnia, arousal and 'jitteriness' early in treatment. The delay in action should be explained carefully to the patient in advance in order to maximise adherence to treatment; likewise, increased arousal early in treatment should be discussed so that the patient understands that a period of persistence may be required before the therapeutic benefits are noticed. This increased arousal early in treatment may be minimised by starting at a low dose and gradually titrating upwards, usually to a high maintenance dose (frequently higher than the maintenance dose for treatment of depression). Treatment should continue for 6–12 months and should only be stopped if the patient has been symptom-free for 3 months, as premature withdrawal may predispose to relapse. More-over, it is important that medication is withdrawn gradually, as sudden cessation may cause a 'discontinuation syndrome', marked by flu-like symptoms, headache, nausea and rebound anxiety symptoms. A suggested prescribing schedule is given in Box 3.3.

Tricyclics

Tricyclic antidepressants with marked serotonergic activity, such as clomipramine, amitriptyline and imipramine, are effective in treating people suffering from anxiety with marked depressive symptoms (of course, SSRIs are also effective in such cases). However, tricyclics tend to have unacceptable side-effects, including blurred vision, constipation and urinary retention. They are also associated with greater lethality in overdose. Therefore, the tricyclics do not have any advantages over

---

> **Box 3.3** Drug treatment in chronic anxiety
>
> **Long-term medication in the treatment of anxiety**
>
> | SSRIs | | |
> |---|---|---|
> | | fluoxetine | (Prozac) |
> | | citalopram | (Cipramil) |
> | | sertraline | (Lustral) |
> | | paroxetine | (Seroxat) |
> | | fluvoxamine | (Faverin) |
> | e.g. | fluoxetine 20–40 mg daily for 3–6 months | |
> | | withdrawn if symptom-free for 3 months. | |

SSRIs and in view of their disadvantages it is recommended that they should only be used where there has been a previous good response or other treatments have failed. A suggested tricyclic, for use in anxiety with obsessive features or associated depression is **Clomipramine**; this may be titrated up from 10 mg daily to a maintenance dose of 150 mg (max. 250 mg daily).

Other drugs

Trazodone

Another drug which may be useful in the long-term treatment of *elderly* people with mixed anxiety and depression is **trazodone** (a sedative antidepressant), which may be titrated up from 50 mg daily to a maintenance dose of 300 mg daily (it is recommended that reference is made to the British National Formulary for current dosing schedules). Monoamine oxidase inhibitors (MAOIs) have also been used to control symptoms of anxiety, but they are best used under specialist supervision.

Beta-blockers

Beta-blockers (beta-adrenergic antagonists) do not affect psychological symptoms such as worry, tension and fear, but they do reduce autonomic symptoms such as palpitations, sweating and tremor. They do not reduce non-autonomic symptoms such as muscle tension. Beta-blockers are therefore indicated for patients with predominantly somatic symptoms and this may in turn prevent the onset of worry and fear.

Patients with predominantly psychological symptoms may obtain no benefit, particularly as beta-blockers may produce disturbed sleep and dreams. Finally, drugs such as **propranolol** may be indicated for the amelioration of performance anxiety (i.e. anxiety associated with performing a particular task) but are not effective in the long-term treatment of generalised anxiety.

Buspirone

Buspirone is an azapirone derivative which acts as an agonist, at presynaptic 5-hydroxytryptamine (5-HT-1α) inhibitory autoreceptors, to lower serotonin levels in the short-term; it is thought that repeated buspirone administration may desensitise neuronal 5-HT auto-inhibition, thereby potentiating serotonin production in the long-term. Although buspirone was developed during the 1980s, it has only recently gained a licence for the treatment of anxiety. It is effective in treating generalised anxiety, but may take up to 2 weeks (in contrast to benzodiazepines which act immediately). In addition, there is little evidence that buspirone causes dependence or tolerance, and withdrawal reactions are not usually problematic. It does not alleviate the symptoms of benzodiazepine withdrawal, so if given as an alternative to benzodiazepine therapy, the latter should be tapered in the usual manner. The adverse effects of buspirone include nausea, dizziness and headache; rarely it may cause palpitations, chest pain, dry mouth, fatigue and sweating. These points are summarised in Box 3.4.

Drug treatment of refractory anxiety

Where a patient fails to respond to any of the conventional drug treatments outlined above, it will be necessary to review the diagnosis; physical causes of symptoms should again be sought (e.g. thyrotoxicosis, cardiac arrhythmia, phaeochromocytoma) before commencing a new drug regime. Moreover, where anxiety symptoms persist or the patient deteriorates despite active treatment, it is recommended that specialist consultation be sought.

Managing benzodiazepine use

Benzodiazepines are seemingly ubiquitous in the practice of modern medicine, and their over-use in the past has occasioned strong public concern. This has resulted in a marked swing amongst medical

---

Box 3.4 Buspirone

- **Action:** agonist at presynaptic 5-HT-1α inhibitory autoreceptors
- **Indication:** adjunctive or short-term monotherapy in anxiety disorder
- **Dose:** 5 mg TDS initially, increased as necessary to 10 mg TDS (max. 15 mg daily)
- **Delay:** may take up to 2 weeks to produce clinical benefit
- **Dependence:** little evidence of tolerance or withdrawal
- **Adverse effects:** nausea, dizziness and headache; rarely palpitations, chest pain, dry mouth, fatigue and sweating

---

practitioners away from using such drugs. Whilst a profligate tendency to prescribe benzodiazepines should clearly be censured, they do nonetheless retain a useful place in the therapeutic armamentarium. It is because of the important role that these drugs have played in public, medical and legal life that there follows a special section on the appropriate use of benzodiazepines.

Although there has been a tendency to prescribe these drugs to almost anyone with stress-related symptoms, unhappiness or minor physical disease, their use in many situations is unjustified. Markus *et al.* (1989) suggest that the use of benzodiazepines as anxiolytics should be restricted to four clinical situations.

1 When the precipitating cause of anxiety is no longer present and the patient is trapped in a vicious circle of self-perpetuating anxiety leading to traumatic symptoms which then cause more anxiety. If anxiety management has failed, a short (2–4 weeks) course of benzodiazepine may break the vicious circle so that it does not become re-established when the medication is discontinued.

2 When anxiety is preventing people from doing important things such as attending dental appointments, starting a new job or travelling for a holiday, a few intermittent doses of a benzodiazepine will often overcome this obstacle and restore confidence.

3 People who are agoraphobic are often afraid to leave home for fear

that a panic attack will occur while they are out and they will be unable to do anything to relieve it. The provision of a small supply 'for emergencies only' will give them added security so much so that the drug may be carried but never taken.

4 Finally, benzodiazepines may be used in treating alcohol withdrawal. The recommended drug is chlordiazepoxide given in a reducing regime e.g. 20 mg QDS reducing over 3–4 days to 5 mg QDS (see British National Formulary for current dosing schedules). Alcohol detoxification usually takes place in acute medical wards, but planned detoxification may be carried out in the home as long as there is adequate supervision (i.e. a community nurse calling at least daily).

In particular, benzodiazepines should not be used to treat depression, phobic or obsessional states or chronic psychosis. In bereavement, psychological adjustment may be inhibited by benzodiazepines. Dependence is particularly likely in patients with a history of alcoholism or drug abuse and in patients with marked personality disorders. The problems associated with benzodiazepines are listed in Box 3.5.

Box 3.5 Problems associated with benzodiazepines

- benzodiazepine dependence
- over-sedation and psychomotor impairment
- increased risk of accidents
- adverse effects on mood and behaviour
- adverse effects on sleep
- interaction with alcohol and other drugs
- potential for abuse and overdose
- risks during pregnancy and lactation
- endocrine dysfunction
- sexual dysfunction
- diminished motivation
- lowered sense of competency
- lower self-esteem
- readiness to adopt a sick role

Safe use of benzodiazepines

The Committee on the Safety of Medicines advises that benzodiazepines are indicated for the short-term relief (2–4 weeks only) of anxiety that is severe, i.e. disabling, subjecting the individual to unacceptable distress, occurring alone or in association with insomnia, short-term psycho-somatic, organic or psychotic illness. In their view the use of benzodiazepines to treat short-term mild anxiety is inappropriate and unsuitable. Benzodiazepines should be used to treat insomnia only when it is severe, disabling or subjecting the individual to extreme distress.

Diazepam, alprazolam, bromazepam, chlordiazepoxide, clobazam, clorazepate and medazepam have a sustained action. Shorter acting compounds such as lorazepam and oxazepam may be preferred in patients with hepatic impairment but they carry a greater risk of withdrawal symptoms. Diazepam or lorazepam are very occasionally administered intravenously for the control of severe panic. This route is the most rapid but the procedure is not without risk and should be used only when alternative measures have failed. Intramuscular diazepam has no advantage over the oral route.

Adverse effects. Benzodiazepine adverse effects are generally mild but include drowsiness, confusion, short-term memory impairment and ataxia. Aggression, ranging from talkativeness and excitement to aggressive and antisocial acts, sometimes occurs but adjustment of the dose usually results in improvement. Increased anxiety and perceptual disorders are other paradoxical effects. Cumulative hangover effects can occur, particularly with compounds with long elimination half-lives, especially in the elderly and in those with impaired hepatic function. The interaction of benzodiazepines and alcohol must be borne in mind and brought to the attention of patients using mechanical machinery or driving.

Patients are more likely to become dependent on benzodiazepines if they are prescribed for a chronic condition and if the patient's personality is characterised by unstable personal relationships and anxiety. Those most at risk are women with social problems and previous users of psychotropic drugs. It is usually easier for patients to stop a short course of such treatment if an underlying problem has been resolved. Sometimes patients may experience withdrawal symptoms while taking benzodiazepines; this reflects the development of tolerance. The main symptom of this is anxiety, which tends to be resolved in 2–4 weeks but occasionally persists. This tends to occur more often with potent rapidly eliminated benzodiazepines, which when used for insomnia can result in daytime withdrawal symptoms as the drug level falls. This may lead to the patient requesting daytime medication to avoid withdrawal effects.

Benzodiazepines and the elderly

Box 3.6 Special considerations in elderly people prescribed benzodiazepines

- cumulative effect of longer acting drugs
- potentiation of other psychotropic drugs and alcohol
- renal impairment
- hepatic impairment
- co-administration of drugs such as cimetidine may raise benzodiazepine levels
- respiratory depression
- drowsiness leading to falls and fractures
- memory impairment and paradoxical aggressive reactions

Benzodiazepine policy in general practice

Beaumont (1991) reiterated the recommendation that GPs should have a clearly defined benzodiazepine policy. A proportion of benzodiazepine prescriptions are written for long-term users and it is important to reach explicit agreement with the patient concerned about the duration and dose of such a prescription, as well as the risks and benefits. There is less difficulty with long-term use involving intermittent or occasional dose regimens. Long-term continuous use needs to be discouraged. There may be justification for such use in patients with chronic severe anxiety disorders and in some elderly patients, bearing in mind pharmacokinetic issues.

Dependence and withdrawal. The benzodiazepine withdrawal syndrome is relatively delayed in onset (although less so with short-acting compounds) but some symptoms may continue for weeks or months. The characteristics of benzodiazepine withdrawal syndrome are shown in Box 3.7. These symptoms may be similar to the original complaint and encourage further prescribing.

Box 3.7 Characteristics of benzodiazepine withdrawal syndrome

- anxiety
- depression
- insomnia
- nausea
- loss of appetite
- loss of body weight
- tremor
- perspiration
- depersonalisation
- perceptual disturbance
- intolerance of loud noise, bright light or touch
- visual hallucinations
- confusion
- epileptic seizures

Protocol. A suggested protocol for patients unable to reduce existing benzodiazepines is shown in Box 3.8. These patients tend to be women in the latter half of life who have been taking benzodiazepines in modest doses (10 mg per day) for several years. The patient must want to stop benzodiazepines and should be educated about the risks and benefits of stopping medication. The patient should be psychiatrically stable, relatively unconcerned about symptoms and there should be no currently pressing social problems or physical ill-health (or any foreseen in the near future).

Existing benzodiazepines can be withdrawn in steps ranging from a tenth to a quarter of the daily dose every fortnight. The time needed for withdrawal can vary from one to several months and withdrawal symptoms may persist for a year or more.

Regular supportive counselling is probably helpful and may take place in groups within general practice or in self-help groups organised within general practice or in self-help groups organised within the statutory, voluntary or private sectors. Beta-blockers have a minor role in the management of benzodiazepine withdrawal but should be tried if other measures fail. Antidepressants should be used if clinical

> **Box 3.8** Suggested protocol for reducing benzodiazepine use
>
> - transfer patient to equivalent daily dose of diazepam, preferably taken at night
> - reduce diazepam dose in fortnightly steps of 2 or 2.5 mg
> - if withdrawal symptoms occur maintain this dose until symptoms improve
> - reduce dose further if necessary in small fortnightly steps
> - it is better to reduce too slowly rather than too quickly
> - stop completely
>
> *Note*: Diazepam 5 mg is approximately equivalent to chlordiazepoxide 5 mg, lorazepam 500 µg, nitrazepam 5 mg, oxazepam 15 mg and temazepam 10 mg.

depression is present; their precise role in this context remains under review. Anti-psychotics and buspirone, which may aggravate withdrawal symptoms, should be avoided. Clonidine and carbamazepine may have a place in management where there is some likelihood of epileptic seizures.

A small proportion of patients can 'just stop', but for the majority, the outcome of benzodiazepine withdrawal is variable and the long-term course probably resembles that of a relapsing and remitting condition.

Patients who raise special difficulties or who fail to respond should be referred to specialist units dealing with benzodiazepine withdrawal. Local psychiatric units should have the relevant information available.

Summary of drug treatment

In summarising the drug treatment of GAD it should always be emphasised that pharmacological approaches alone are unlikely to produce enduring benefit. Although drug treatment and psychological treatment may be of equal benefit in isolation they appear to have a synergistic effect when combined, and there is increasing evidence that combined pharmacological and psychological treatment reduces the rate of relapse following discontinuation of medication. This clearly has important implications not only for long-term costs (reducing future consultations, etc.), but also promises a much more positive outlook for the individual in terms of future morbidity (and indeed mortality, which has been shown to be increased in chronic anxiety states). The main points of drug treatment for GAD are summarised in Box 3.9.

Box 3.9 Drug treatment of GAD

- **Short-term**: Diazepam 2–5 mg TDS (max. 10 mg TDS) for 2–4 weeks, only if severe symptoms
- **Long-term**: SSRI, e.g. paroxetine titrated in 10 mg increments fortnightly to 40 mg daily. Gradual withdrawal after 3 months asymptomatic period
- **Adjunctive therapy**: Buspirone 5–10 mg TDS (max. 15 mg TDS) as adjunct to long-term therapy refractory anxiety (may be used as short-term monotherapy in patients naïve to benzodiazepines)

Matching agent to patient

The 'Anxiety Decision Tree' as shown in Figure 3.1 is a simple to follow algorithm for the management of patients presenting with anxiety symptoms. It is based on research findings, but is not intended to be prescriptive; as always the clinician and patient should arrive at the treatment plan most suitable for each given situation, and a good therapeutic alliance between patient and therapist remains the most valuable component of treatment.

In selecting an appropriate drug for the treatment of anxiety disorders, it should be borne in mind that there is marginal difference in efficacy between the various SSRIs. Hence the decision as to which SSRI to use should take into consideration not only the existing clinical evidence base concerning each anxiety syndrome (as summarised in Table 3.1), but also factors such as individual patient tolerability and side-effect profile. Hence it may be necessary to try more than one drug before identifying that which is most suitable for a given patient. A recent review of the scientific literature (den Boer, 1999) provides a convenient summary of evidence-based indications for the various SSRIs in anxiety-related disorders.

Psychological treatment of anxiety

This section covers the general psychological principles and procedures used in the treatment of anxiety disorders. Particular psychological

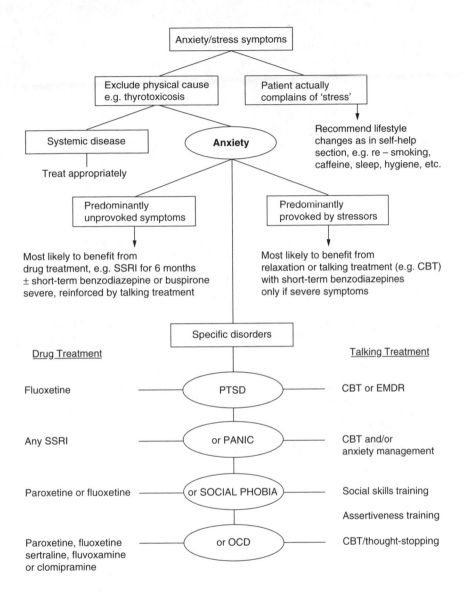

Anxiety/stress symptoms

Exclude physical cause
e.g. thyrotoxicosis

Patient actually
complains of 'stress'

Recommend lifestyle
changes as in self-help
section, e.g. re – smoking,
caffeine, sleep, hygiene, etc.

Systemic disease

Anxiety

Treat appropriately

Predominantly
unprovoked symptoms

Predominantly
provoked by stressors

Most likely to benefit from
drug treatment, e.g. SSRI for 6 months
± short-term benzodiazepine or buspirone
severe, reinforced by talking treatment

Most likely to benefit from
relaxation or talking treatment (e.g. CBT)
with short-term benzodiazepines
only if severe symptoms

Specific disorders

Drug Treatment

Talking Treatment

Fluoxetine — PTSD — CBT or EMDR

Any SSRI — or PANIC — CBT and/or
anxiety management

Paroxetine or fluoxetine — or SOCIAL PHOBIA — Social skills training

Assertiveness training

Paroxetine, fluoxetine — or OCD — CBT/thought-stopping
sertraline, fluvoxamine
or clomipramine

Key: SSRI   Selective Serotonin Reuptake Inhibitor
       CBT   Cognitive-Behaviour Therapy
       EMDR   Eye Movement Desensitisation Retraining

Figure 3.1 The anxiety treatment tree, an algorithm for the management of anxiety disorders.

Table 3.1 SSRIs in anxiety disorders

	OCD	Panic	Social phobia	PTSD	GAD
Paroxetine	~ +	~ +	~ +		
Fluoxetine	~ +	~ +	~	~ +	+/-
Citalopram		~ +	~		
Sertraline	~ +	~ +	~	~	
Fluvoxamine	~ +	~ +	~ +	~	+/-

OCD, obsessive compulsive disorder; PTSD, post traumatic stress disorder; GAD, generalised anxiety disorder; ~, open data; +, controlled study.
Adapted from den Boer, 1999.

techniques specific to each anxiety disorder are discussed in the appropriate chapters, along with relevant psychological models to explain each disorder. Self-help material, including descriptions of many of the anxiety-management techniques discussed, is included in Chapter 9. Appendix 2 includes recording and information sheets which the GP can copy and give out to patients.

Anxiety-management training

Anxiety management aims to help patients cope more effectively with anxiety symptoms, and includes a combination of:

- identifying anxiety-provoking thoughts and situations
- formal training in relaxation skills
- generating self-reassuring instructions to promote confidence
- deliberately creating anxiety-provoking images and thoughts, which are brought under control by replacing them with coping images and thoughts.

Learning relaxation skills helps the patient feel less anxious, more able to control anxiety when it does occur and enables patients to attempt more activities (instructions for progressive muscular relaxation can be found in Chapter 9). Focusing on, and 'catastrophising' about, symptoms serves to maintain anxiety symptoms, therefore distraction is a useful short-term skill to teach the patient. If the patient feels more able to control upsetting or catastrophic thoughts they will be more likely to control the vicious cycle of anxiety. Such techniques are usually presented and practised in anxiety-management groups, but can quickly be outlined by the GP to patients who appear articulate and motivated to develop skills necessary to help themselves. Such self-help strategies are explained in more detail in Chapter 9, and patient recording and information sheets are provided in Appendix 2.

Cognitive-behaviour therapy

Behavioural treatment is well established and has proven efficacy for anxiety disorders. It includes **exposure** treatment with **systematic desensitisation**; these procedures are discussed below. More recently, therapists have begun to focus attention on the **cognitive component** of anxiety disorders and the role that the patient's thoughts, beliefs and expectations have on the aetiology and maintenance of their symptoms. The most impressive work done by cognitive therapists so far has been in the treatment of depression. The expansion of behaviour therapy to include aspects of the patient's 'thought-life' is labelled **cognitive-behaviour therapy (CBT)** and has become the mainstay of psychological treatment for anxiety disorders. The patient's cognitions (thoughts, beliefs, mental images) about their fears and associated symptoms are elicited and the therapist aids in the modification and 'testing out' of harmful or erroneous cognitions.

Table 3.2 outlines the CBT interventions recommended for each anxiety disorder. Some of these measures need specialist advice or training, but many are well within the capabilities of the GP – skills and time being available. Increasingly, greater numbers of GPs are gaining training and expertise in CBT for psychological disorders. Practice manuals are available (Carnwath and Miller, 1986; France and Robson, 1986; Greenberger and Padesky, 1995).

Rationale and education

Early in treatment it is useful to provide patients with written information regarding the nature of anxiety, including the symptoms and their relationship to adrenaline (the 'fight/flight' hormone), their

Table 3.2 Recommended CBT interventions

Anxiety disorder	Common behaviours and cognitions	Interventions
Generalised anxiety, Chapter 3	what if ... happens? overestimate danger, underestimate coping ability belief of vulnerability	identify triggers look for evidence develop coping plans change core beliefs
Agoraphobia and other phobias, Chapter 4	specific situational fears, avoidance	identify specific fear look for evidence develop a coping plan exposure to fear with practice in coping
Panic disorder, Chapter 5	catastrophic fears related to physical or mental sensations	identify specific fears exposure to sensations develop alternative explanation for sensations experiments to test fears
Post-traumatic stress disorder, Chapter 7	thoughts regarding meaning of the trauma vulnerability beliefs flashbacks guilt and shame	identify distressing meaning of trauma look for survivorship meaning in trauma develop coping plans evaluate maladaptive beliefs
Obsessive-compulsive disorder, Chapter 8	intrusive thoughts are dangerous thinking things makes them happen	identify beliefs regarding danger and responsibility test beliefs about obsessive thoughts exposure to fears response prevention

possible biological origin and function, reassuring them that the associated autonomic changes are not detrimental to their physical health or to their mental sanity. This information is tailored to the particular needs of each patient.

As with CBT for all manner of psychological disorders, the initial objective is to present the rationale underlying treatment to the patient, ensuring that they have a good understanding of the model on which intervention is based. It is helpful to use a simplified version of the psychological models illustrated in this text to explain the process, inserting details pertinent to each patient's situation.

Behavioural aspects of treatment

Exposure therapy

Exposure therapy is extremely beneficial for patients with phobias, panic or compulsive rituals. It can also work well as a form of self-help if carried out systematically. The main principle is to enable the patient to identify and return to the main stimulus or frightening situation which has been avoided and to stay in contact with that stimulus for at least 30 minutes per day (preferably 1–2 hours). With daily repetition, the patient's fear and their desire to avoid the situation gradually disappear with habituation. Most people require only simple explanation and a few hours' practise of the techniques described. In more complex or severe cases, up to 20 hours of treatment may be required to enable the patient to come into contact with the feared situation and either have limited anxiety or be able to cope. In such cases, however, it is usually a mental health nurse who will provide the majority of treatment.

The main weapon in the therapist's armamentarium against excessive avoidance behaviour is the introduction of planned and systematic exposure exercises. To some extent, exposure also functions as a 'behavioural test' in that the person's maladaptive cognitions are challenged and disconfirmed during exposure. Avoidance maintains the patient's negative beliefs, hence it is important that the therapist encourages patients to enter into situations previously avoided in order to 'test out' their fears. Do the things they are afraid will happen actually occur? Patients are encouraged to expose themselves to feared situations repeatedly and in a graded fashion, whilst relaxed (see section on 'fear hierarchies' in Chapter 4). In addition, patients' predictions of what they think will happen are compared with the real outcome. Patients are asked to state, not only their predicted fear level (e.g. 70%) but also anticipated catastrophies ('I will have a heart attack/faint/make a fool of myself'). Often patients accurately predict experienced fear but their predictions of anticipated catastrophies are rarely correct.

The GP is there to instruct the patient how to treat themselves, it is for the patient to undertake the exposure exercise themselves. The help of a relative or friend as 'co-therapist' may be crucial in gaining compliance and maintaining motivation, and only in the more chronic and entrenched cases is extensive face-to-face professional therapy required. As already mentioned, this would normally be carried out by a mental health nurse. Some examples of the use of exposure are outlined in Boxes 3.10 and 3.11.

Exposure to the feared stimulus, situation or image will understandably provoke an anxiety response. It is therefore crucial to the success of this procedure to help the individual plan how they will cope with this. Various anxiety-management strategies are taught and practised to competence prior to exposure. Exposure-evoked anxiety

---

Box 3.10   Non-drug treatment of compulsive rituals

- People with compulsive rituals are encouraged to enter into situations that make them feel uncomfortable and make them want to wash, check or tidy up. They are asked to resist these urges until they die down, which may take an hour or more. This is termed **response prevention.**

- For example, when calm, a patient is asked to touch a dirty surface that would usually evoke the urge to wash their hands. If allowed to wash their hands the distress and urge would quickly disappear but would reappear again soon after. Instead, the patient is asked firmly but supportively not to wash for at least an hour. The initial anxiety and urge to wash are intense but gradually subside until the patient is as calm as at the start of the 1–2 hour session.

Box 3.11   Non-drug treatment of agoraphobia

- The patient is encouraged to chose one of their currently avoided activities which they would most like to undertake. The patient then engages in these activities in a graduated manner, for at least an hour at a time, until habituation is achieved and full activity is accomplished.

- It is important to specify exactly, in words, what the particular activity entails so that the patient knows when they have achieved their desired aim. These specific goals should also be relatively achieveable initially, with gradual increments in difficulty accompanying improvements in the patient's skill level.

may be relieved by the '6–second breath', mental distraction from bodily sensations and relaxation (*see* Chapter 9 for further details). The term **reciprocal inhibition** refers to the finding that approaching the feared stimulus in a calm, relaxed state acts to inhibit the physiological fear response. With generalised anxiety, paradoxical instructions are often employed – in which patients may be encouraged to imagine the worst disaster that could befall them in that situation. The patient is enabled to develop a plan of exactly what they could do to cope if 'the worst happened'.

It may be necessary to continue with exposure exercises for weeks or months in order to see improvement in a patient's functioning. During the intervals between consultations, progress with exposure 'experiments' can be monitored by the patient in diary sheets (see Figures 3.2–3.4). Habituation is specific to the particular feared situation to which the patient is exposed and generalisation to other feared situations cannot automatically be expected. It is therefore often necessary for all feared situations to be included in the treatment, but patients will soon be able to independently apply the principles for themselves in many spontaneous fear-provoking situations.

The guiding rules of exposure

Exposure should provoke anxiety. However, patients who employ techniques to control anxiety symptoms during exposure (as detailed in Chapter 9) will move faster up their hierarchy. They will have the skills necessary to deal better with anticipatory anxiety and will be able to apply them to any anxious situation occurring in the future, thus increasing their self-confidence and the active generalisation of these skills.

Research suggests that for maximal effectiveness exposure should be graduated, repeated and prolonged. Practice tasks should be clearly specified by the use of a hierarchy. The first task should be easy enough for the patient to be sure they can attempt it, but sufficient to provoke some anxiety. Tasks which do not provoke anxiety are not useful as they do not provide a context for new learning.

Tasks should be repeated frequently and regularly until they provoke only a little anxiety, prior to proceeding to the next item in the hierarchy. Each task should be prolonged until anxiety levels begin to subside, and progress will be faster the shorter the time interval between tasks. The more patients practise, the quicker they improve.

However, the more complex the disorder, the longer it will take to treat. Eight sessions are usually adequate for the patient to understand

Date: _____

Target: _____
_____
_____

Time: _____

Alone or accompanied: _____

If accompanied, by whom: _____

Anxiety (0–100)   Before: _____

                   During (highest): _____

                   After: _____

Any panics: _____

Comments: _____
_____
_____
_____

Ideas for next target: _____
_____
_____

Figure 3.2 Exposure practice chart.

Date:

Description of task:

For each stage listed, give your rating by circling the cross underneath the number which best describes *how you feel at the time*.
Do the rating *in the situation itself*, NOT later when you think back.

SITUATION	I don't feel at all uncomfortable										I feel the most uncomfortable I have ever felt
	0	10	20	30	40	50	60	70	80	90	100
_____	X	X	X	X	X	X	X	X	X	X	X
_____	X	X	X	X	X	X	X	X	X	X	X
_____	X	X	X	X	X	X	X	X	X	X	X
_____	X	X	X	X	X	X	X	X	X	X	X
_____	X	X	X	X	X	X	X	X	X	X	X
_____	X	X	X	X	X	X	X	X	X	X	X
_____	X	X	X	X	X	X	X	X	X	X	X
_____	X	X	X	X	X	X	X	X	X	X	X
_____ MINUTES LATER	X	X	X	X	X	X	X	X	X	X	X

Figure 3.3 Recording sheet for a behavioural test/experiment.

Situation	What I predict will happen	Negative thoughts about the situation	What actually happened	Change in thoughts afterwards

Figure 3.4 Monitoring changes in thoughts in response to exposure.

the method and continue applying it for themselves with only minimal help. A summary of exposure treatment is given in Box 3.12.

Box 3.12 Summary of exposure treatment

- employ techniques to control anxiety symptoms during exposure
- deal with anticipatory anxiety prior to attempting exposure tasks
- apply anxiety controlling techniques to any future anxious situations

Hierarchy:

- practice tasks should be clearly specified by the use of a hierarchy
- tasks should be graduated, repeated and prolonged
- each task should be prolonged until anxiety levels begin to subside
- tasks are repeated frequently and regularly until they provoke only a little anxiety
- move onto the next task in the hierarchy

Graded exposure

Exposure can be *in vivo* or imagined (where the patient imagines approaching feared situations). *In vivo* exposure is generally more effective, but exposure through imagination may be a necessary step before the patient feels able to progress to *in vivo* exposure, which is more anxiety provoking.

Exposure can be immediate, direct and full (often termed **flooding**, e.g. an agoraphobic patient taken to Piccadilly Circus on a Saturday afternoon) or be graded **systematic desensitisation** (where the feared situation is approached in graded steps, hierarchically), starting with the least feared element (anxiety rating = 0) and working gradually up to the most feared aspect (anxiety rating = 100). The patient moves onto the next step when they just feel able to manage the last one. Again, graded exposure may begin in imagination and progress to *in vivo*. Modulating factors, such as the presence of a trusted person or distance from the feared object, are considered in order to fill all the steps from 0 to 100. It is important that the hierarchy includes all the feared and avoided objects and situations relevant to that individual. A hierarchy sheet, named 'fear ladder' (*see* Figure 3.5) is provided, with a completed example given in Chapter 4, regarding a fear of heights.

Cognitive aspects of treatment

In addition to behavioural approaches, therapists have begun to focus attention on the **cognitive component** of anxiety. Certain patterns of thinking and specific thought content are more common in particular anxiety disorders and will be covered in the relevant chapters. However, the basic principles of cognitive therapy remain the same; the patient's cognitions relating to their anxiety and associated symptoms are elicited and the therapist aids in the modification and 'testing out' of harmful or erroneous cognitions, thus affecting both their behaviour and thoughts.

Identifying anxious thoughts

In order to modify maladaptive cognitions it is first necessary to identify them. To this end, it is useful to obtain from the patient a detailed description of a recent anxious situation, be it a panic attack, compulsive ritual or social situation. It is particularly important to focus on the thoughts or mental images experienced during the episode and any links with specific bodily symptoms. For example, in Chapter 5 (Panic attacks), we shall see that breathlessness and a pounding heart often trigger thoughts of an impending heart attack.

It is important to help the patient identify their specific fears, apprehensions and negative thoughts, as well as their symptoms and possible triggers for anxiety. It may take some time before they become familiar with identifying their particular thoughts and catastrophic interpretations for their symptoms. This can be facilitated by the use of thoughts diaries as discussed further in Chapter 9. A thoughts diary, Figure 3.6, is provided here.

Mood shifts during sessions are particularly useful sources of automatic thoughts. During discussions about activities avoided or fearful situations, the therapist notices when the patient becomes tense and anxious and asks 'What went through your mind just then?'

Other methods of eliciting negative thoughts include using imagery or role-play, where patients either relive the emotional event by replaying it in great detail in their 'mind's eye' or by role-playing the situation with the therapist. The patient is encouraged to slowly run the image forward, verbalising what they are feeling and thinking at each stage.

		Rating scale (0–100)
1	______________________________	__________
2	______________________________	__________
3	______________________________	__________
4	______________________________	__________
5	______________________________	__________
6	______________________________	__________
7	______________________________	__________
8	______________________________	__________
9	______________________________	__________
10	______________________________	__________

Ideas to help you construct this hierarchy:

- looking at pictures of the stimulus, or watching films
- think of real-life situations
- watching someone else do it first
- doing things first with someone, then alone
- think of the things that make each task easier or harder – distance from the object, having particular people around, being in new or unfamiliar places

Figure 3.5 Hierarchy/fear ladder.

Thoughts Diary (A–B–C chart)

Date and time	Situation What were you doing? Anyone else there?	Emotions What did you feel? Rate 0–10	Thoughts Use exact words, How much did you believe them? Rate 0–10	Rational response What are your answers to the 'NATs'? How much do you believe them? Rate 0–10

Figure 3.6 Thoughts diary.

Modifying cognitions

Once the patient's anxious thoughts have been identified, a number of techniques are introduced to help the person gain safer and more appropriate interpretations of events. Patients often catastrophise about the outcome of a situation or how others will view them. They are encouraged to generate alternative, more balanced responses to these thoughts. Also at this stage, any worrying bodily sensations are correctly attributed to their own heightened awareness and the physiological effects of anxiety.

The techniques used to modify these thoughts are common to cognitive therapy for other emotional disorders:

- search for alternative explanations
- considering how other people would interpret the situation
- inclusion of otherwise ignored facts
- rejecting misleading 'facts' which are being believed
- trying to estimate the probability that the feared catastrophic event will actually take place.

Box 3.13 Self-questioning: tips for coping with anxiety

- 'What evidence do I have for/against this thought?'
- 'Is there an alternative explanation for the situation?'
- 'How can my new understanding of the effects of anxiety on my body help me explain what's happening?'
- 'How would someone else think about the situation?'
- 'Are you setting yourself an unrealistic standard?'
- 'Are you forgetting relevant facts or focusing only on irrelevant facts?'
- 'Are you thinking in all-or-nothing terms?'
- 'What if it did happen? What would be so bad about that?'
- 'Are you underestimating what you can do to deal with the problem/situation?'
- 'Are you overestimating the probability of a negative event occurring?'

The therapist trains the individual to ask questions of themselves during their episodes of anxiety, the most common of which include those given in Box 3.13.

The use of a thoughts diary will enable them to continue this work outside therapy sessions (*see* Figures 3.4 and 3.6).

Belief ratings, as used in the thoughts diary, are an effective method of monitoring the patient's success in challenging their irrational beliefs and erroneous interpretations. The patient is asked to rate how much they believe a particular identified anxious thought on a scale from 0 – 'I don't believe it at all' to 100 – 'I am absolutely convinced'. Repeated belief ratings can then be used to monitor progress within and between sessions. It is important that the therapist check that treatment has reduced beliefs in real-life feared situations and not just in the clinic.

Preventing relapse

To prevent relapse, towards the end of therapy, the sessions focus on education, self-reliance and anticipating setbacks. The time between sessions is gradually increased. It is anticipated that the patient will take on increasingly more of the planning of sessions to ensure they have a clear grasp of the procedures employed and develop confidence in carrying these out independently. Discussion relates to which skills have been most effective and how they could be adapted to possible future problems. Mention is made of circumstances in which relapse may occur, such as stresses or conflicts, losses or bereavements, episodes of ill health and the introduction of new catastrophic cognitions.

Some patients may find it useful to write out a plan of action if their anxiety disorder should recur. An example for a patient with panic attacks is provided in Chapter 5, Box 5.11.

It is important for the patient to know that they can regain contact for continued help should the problem become unmanageable. 'Booster sessions' are generally successful in maintaining treatment effects over time. For many patients, the mere knowledge that the system remains open is sufficient to provide the security needed to enable them to continue independently.

Appendix 3A

Generalised anxiety – F41.1

Adapted from WHO (1996)

Presenting complaints

The patient may present initially with tension-related physical symptoms (e.g. headache, pounding heart) or with insomnia. Enquiry will reveal prominent anxiety.

Diagnostic features

Multiple symptoms of anxiety or tension:

- mental tension (worry, feeling tense or nervous, poor concentration)
- physical tension (restlessness, headaches, tremors, inability to relax)
- physical arousal (dizziness, sweating, fast or pounding heart, dry mouth, stomach pains).

Symptoms may last for months and recur often. They are often triggered by stressful events in those with a chronic tendency to worry.

Differential diagnosis

- If low or sad mood is prominent, see *Depression – F32#.*
- If sudden attacks of unprovoked anxiety are present, see *Panic disorder – F41.0.*
- If fear and avoidance of specific situations are present, see *Phobic disorders – F40.*
- If heavy alcohol or drug use is present, see *Alcohol-use disorders – F10* and *Drug-use disorders – F11#.*
- Certain physical conditions (thyrotoxicosis) or medications (methyl xanthines, beta-agonists) may cause symptoms.

Generalised anxiety – F41.1: management guidelines

Essential information for patient and family

- Stress and worry have both physical and mental effects.

- Learning skills to reduce the effects of stress (not sedative medication) is the most effective relief.

Counselling of patient and family

- Encourage the patient to practise daily relaxation methods to reduce physical symptoms of tension.

- Encourage the patient to engage in pleasurable activities and exercise, and to resume activities that have been helpful in the past.

- Identifying and challenging exaggerated worries can reduce anxiety symptoms.

- Identify exaggerated worries or pessimistic thoughts (e.g. when daughter is 5 minutes late from school, patient worries that she may have had an accident).

- Discuss ways to challenge these exaggerated worries when they occur (e.g. when the patient starts to worry about the daughter, the patient could tell him/herself, 'I am starting to be caught up in worry again. My daughter is only a few minutes late and should be home soon. I won't call the school to check unless she's an hour late')

  - Structured problem-solving methods can help patients to manage current life problems or stresses that contribute to anxiety symptoms.

- Identify events that trigger excessive worry (e.g. a young woman presents with worry, tension, nausea and insomnia. These symptoms began after her son was diagnosed with asthma. Her anxiety worsens when he has asthma episodes).

- Discuss what the patient is doing to manage this situation. Identify and reinforce things that are working.

- Identify some specific actions that the patient can take in the next few weeks, such as:

- meet with nurse/doctor/health professionals to learn about the course and management of asthma
- discuss concerns with parents of other asthmatic children
- write down a plan for management of asthma episodes
- regular physical exercise is often helpful.

Medication

Medication is a secondary treatment in the management of generalised anxiety. It may be used, however, if significant anxiety symptoms persist despite counselling.

- Anti-anxiety medication (e.g. diazepam 5–10 mg at night) may be used for no longer than 2 weeks. Longer term use may lead to dependence and is likely to result in the return of symptoms when discontinued.

- Beta-blockers may help control physical symptoms.

- Antidepressant drugs may be helpful (especially if symptoms of depression are present) and do not lead to dependence or rebound symptoms. For details, see *Depression – F32#.*

Specialist consultation

Consultation may be helpful if anxiety is severe.

4
Agoraphobia and other phobias

Phobia is defined as an irrational fear leading to avoidance of a particular situation or object. In contrast to GAD, considered in Chapter 3, phobic anxiety arises in the context of the feared object or situation, and the subject may become anxious just thinking about or anticipating a situation. The phobias are generally categorised into fear of busy places (agoraphobia), fear of social interaction (social phobia) and specific fears (e.g. of spiders – arachnophobia). Each of these phobic disorders will be discussed prior to a discussion of psychological models and CBT for phobias.

Agoraphobia

Definition

Agoraphobia does not mean fear of open spaces (although such a fear can occur). This often surprises the uninitiated and the confusion may be simply clarified by understanding the origins of the term. **Agora** is Greek for 'market' and the predominantly feared situation in agoraphobia is the busy, crowded atmosphere of public places such as shops, or indeed market places. Traditionally it was the homemaker who required regular use of shops, and a fear of going out would keep them at home. This gave rise to the term 'housebound housewife' syndrome, and in fact the majority of sufferers today are married women.

Epidemiology

Agoraphobia accounts for approximately 60% of phobias, and about two-thirds of sufferers are women. The prevalence varies across studies using different diagnostic tools, but one recent estimate using the

Anxiety Screening Questionnaire (ASQ-15) gave a point prevalence of 1.5% for agoraphobia (WHO, 1994).

Aetiology

The aetiology of phobias has considerable overlap with the aetiology of anxiety. The main difference, however, is that with phobias the anxiety is situation specific and not generalised. It is likely that this clinical distinction reflects subtle differences in the underlying biological mechanisms, but specific neuropathology remains to be fully described.

Biological

The biological aspects of anxiety symptoms have been dealt with in Chapter 1 and will be summarised briefly here. Anxiety and arousal symptoms are associated with increased activity of the locus coeruleus, which lies in the rostral pons adjacent to the cerebral aqueduct. It is the major noradrenergic centre of the brain, and has extensive efferents to the limbic system. The rostral PAG mediates a 'fight' response and the caudal PAG (the site of the locus coeruleus) produces a 'flight' response; the latter is also richly innervated by an inhibitory input of GABA neurones.

Genetic

Agoraphobia has been the most extensively studied phobia, probably reflecting the fact that it is the most common type of phobia. Relatives of patients with agoraphobia are at increased risk not only for agoraphobia, but also for other phobias (whereas relatives of patients with panic disorder were only at increased risk of panic).

This suggests that there exist population groups with either a tendency for phobias or a tendency for panic, with an overlapping sub-group who inherit a tendency to both panic and phobia (as is seen, for example in agoraphobia with panic attacks).

In phobic anxiety, increased noradrenergic activity from the locus coeruleus is presumed only to occur during exposure to certain stimuli, and it is likely that psychological factors mediate the anxiety response. In other words, exposure to *perceived* threat (even when there is none) produces an expectation of danger, resulting in a physiological response of arousal. This concept invokes the 'learned' model of phobias, which is discussed below in the context of psychological causes.

Psychological

The primary assumption of all behavioural accounts of phobias is that such fear reactions are learned. Despite much clinical and research interest in this area over many decades, one single theory to account for all phobias has not yet been identified. Several behavioural mechanisms have been proposed: avoidance conditioning, modelling (also known as vicarious conditioning – when the fear is learned by observing fear in others without coming into direct contact with the stimulus themselves) and operant conditioning.

In the case of agoraphobia, the model of classical conditioning can be used to account for the clinical features of the disorder. A subject encounters a 'neutral' environment such as a shopping arcade (NS – neutral stimulus) and happens to experience symptoms of panic (UR – unconditioned response) in response to a fleeting palpitation (US – unconditioned stimulus). If anxiety symptoms are very severe they may become associated with the environment (CS – conditioned stimulus) after only one pairing (i.e. single trial learning) and as a result shopping is thereafter associated with panic or anxiety and therefore avoided.

Fear/avoidance conditioning is a form of learning whereby a new association develops between a previously neutral stimulus and one's subjective fear and related physiological responses to it. For example, a child playing with a pet dog (the neutral stimulus) may annoy it and get bitten. The child understandably responds with fear and distress, and learns to avoid dogs in the future. Many people become intensely afraid of driving a car after a serious accident or of descending stairs after a bad fall. However, patients may not always be able to describe one single such traumatic event occurring to date the onset of the disorder. The phobic response often builds up gradually, resulting from repeated frightening experiences, often occurring at times of stress or high arousal, when fear responses are more easily learned. Avoidance of the stimulus is thus negatively reinforced by the subsequent reduction in the fear response in the absence of the feared object or situation.

The learning of phobic responses by observing others is known as **vicarious conditioning** and operates via the concept of social learning. Phobias may develop by seeing the fear response elicited in someone else by a stimulus, or simply by their verbal reports of ensuing disastrous consequences.

Phobias relating to certain objects or situations may become conditioned when avoidance is positively reinforced. For example, school refusal in a child may be maintained by favourable consequences, such as staying close to a parent. Such a mechanism can be understood by **operant conditioning** principles, whereby a certain behaviour is maintained and made more likely because of the payoff provided by the environment. This is not to neglect the fact that the lives of many phobics become severely limited through their compelling need to avoid harmless situations.

People with phobias react to feared stimuli in three ways: **physiologically** derived anxiety symptoms include sensations associated with panic and may precipitate full-blown attacks (a different pattern of symptoms is present in blood or injury phobics, when there is a sudden fall in heart rate and fainting); **behavioural** symptoms comprise the 'fight or flight' response; **subjective** symptoms include catastrophic thoughts (e.g. 'The birds may attack me and peck out my eyes', 'I may make a fool of myself') and emotions such as shame, embarrassment, anger and fear. By definition, phobic fear is disproportional to the danger presented and reactions such as avoidance and hypervigilance are clearly inappropriate. Figure 4.1 illustrates how the reactions to symptoms maintain the phobia by creating vicious circles that perpetuate fear.

As explained in previous chapters, avoidance serves to maintain anxiety by preventing the patient from entering the feared situation and thereby learning that it is not in fact dangerous and that they can cope. Other important maintaining factors include the patient's interpretations of their symptomatology ('I'm going to faint'), or about the feared consequences of the situation ('I'll get bitten', 'Nobody will speak to me'), and loss of confidence in their ability to deal with the situation. External factors also play a part; reinforcement and over-protection by family members prevents them facing up to the subject of their fears. In the effective treatment of people with phobias, the precise identification of maintaining factors is crucial.

Natural history

Agoraphobia usually *arises* between the ages of 15 and 35, but established *cases* are commonest between 25 and 44 years of age. Onset frequently occurs after the subject has experienced marked anxiety (commonly a panic attack) in a public place, and this is followed by a period of avoidance of similar places (*see* Box 4.1). This condition tends to pursue one of two courses. On the one hand, it may resolve

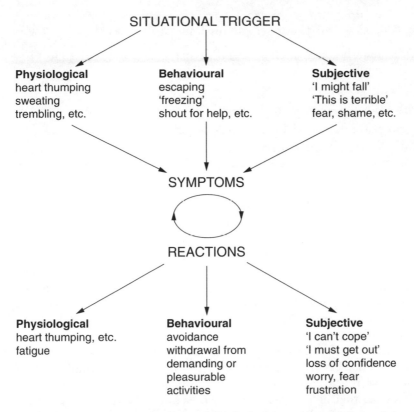

Figure 4.1 A vicious circle model of phobic anxiety (adapted from Hawton *et al.*, 1992).

spontaneously, in patients coming to the attention of specialists 20% experience spontaneous remission, suggesting that many more cases in the community, i.e. not coming into contact with specialists, may undergo limited periods of agoraphobia followed by long periods of remission. On the other hand, if the avoidance becomes generalised to all settings outside the home the course is likely to be unremitting, leading to the 'housebound' syndrome, which may persist for many years. Thus, agoraphobia tends to run either a chronic or a fluctuating course.

Clinical features

The very nature of agoraphobia mitigates against presenting outside the home, and many cases are initially seen by professionals within the home

---

Box 4.1   General points regarding agoraphobia

- 60% of phobic patients seen by psychiatrists suffer from agoraphobia
- 66% are female
- most develop symptoms between 15 and 35 years of age
- term also often used for fear of shopping and crowds
- other non-phobic symptoms are common (generalised anxiety, panic attacks, depression, obsessions, depersonalisation)

---

setting. People with severe, chronic agoraphobia are predominantly housebound (*see* the case example in Box 4.2) and if sorties from home are made at all they are only accomplished with great effort and in the presence of supportive company. In some cases even reminders of the outside world are excluded so that windows remain closed and curtains drawn, doors tightly shut and lights dimmed, the hapless sufferer limited to the joyless existence of a prisoner in their own home. They are fully aware of the unwanted limitations their condition brings and of the unreasonableness of their fears. Family members who once sought to entice the subject outdoors, often at the cost of emotional outbursts and bitter arguments, become wearied in their efforts and eventually submit to an endless round of cosseting behaviours unwittingly calculated to restrict further their loved one's already miserable lifestyle. Typically the disorder is chronic and the associated impairment is severe.

The fears experienced in agoraphobia lead to a particular pattern of dependence upon help from outside and avoidance of normal social activities, resulting in social constriction. The pattern might begin with the fear of a certain shop, but spreads steadily to involve the shopping area of the town and then even to shops in the neighbourhood, culminating in a fear of leaving home.

There are many situations which evoke agoraphobic avoidance, but the most common include: crowded town centres, and particularly indoor shopping centres; supermarkets, especially checkout queues; theatres and cinemas, unless sitting in an aisle seat; and most forms of public transport – such as buses, trains and lifts together with queuing for any of these.

Most people with agoraphobia find that being accompanied in any of these feared situations reduces the dread beforehand and terror once there. Some are supported by a spouse, parent or understanding friend, but many also find that the presence even of young children may permit a trip which would be impossible alone. In this respect a dog, a pram or shopping trolley can be beneficial, and some patients find that they can drive their cars to places which they could not visit on foot.

Some patients give a very clear account of the incident which seemed to start off the pattern, even though this may have occurred many years previously. Such an episode often has all the hallmarks of a panic attack and may have arisen apparently without reason, perhaps whilst on holiday or during normal routine activities. A story of particular stress at the time of onset is sometimes elicited.

Associated features

Although there are no actual percentages available, agoraphobia is very frequently asssociated with panic attacks, at least in its early stages. Clearly, if situations are avoided which characteristically provoke cued panic attacks then such attacks will be minimised, and may be absent altogether in housebound agoraphobia. Other features commonly seen in agoraphobia are depression, which is usually secondary to the phobia, and obsessional symptoms, which may reflect an underlying predisposition or premorbid personality trait. Agoraphobia may also be complicated by alcohol misuse, as described in the case in Box 4.2.

Box 4.2   Case example

Mrs A is a 40-year-old mother of three who is married and works as a housewife. For the last 7 years she has been unable to leave the house on her own. Just the thought of leaving the house made her extremely anxious. She coped by enlisting the help of her children and unemployed husband, who would run errands and do the shopping. Her last venture out of the home was 18 months ago when she attended her mother's funeral; she had to be coaxed by family members to go and then had to leave the gathering early. Recently her youngest child entered school and her husband started working again, which left Mrs A without any means of coping throughout the day. As a result she felt increasingly that she was a failure and began to drink several glasses of sherry during the day. When her husband discovered this he restricted the alcohol in the house and shortly afterwards Mrs A agreed to a home visit by the family doctor.

Presentation

Patients do not usually present to their doctor in the surgery or out-patients department, for reasons already discussed. Often a crisis intervenes, such as severe depression or alcohol problems secondary to agoraphobia, which prompts the individual or a relative to seek medical help, resulting in a home visit by the GP. If specialist referral is made (as usually happens in housebound cases of agoraphobia) the psychiatrists will also normally assess the patient in their own home.

Assessment

Assessment of patients with agoraphobia is frequently carried out in the patient's home. This has a number of advantages, apart from the fact that it may be the *only* way of assessing such patients. Firstly, it provides a unique opportunity to observe the patient within their home environment, allowing judgements to be made about how well the patient is coping, and how limited their lifestyle is. Secondly, it usually permits additional information to be gleaned from at least one other friend or relative. Thirdly, it may enhance the doctor–patient relationship, allowing a strong therapeutic alliance to be established earlier than it might be within the 'doctor's territory'. Fourthly, it allows judgements to be made concerning the degree to which family members might be reinforcing the avoidant behaviour. Fifthly, it allows possible identification of family members who may act as 'therapy facilitators'. Finally, a home visit enables the doctor (or nurse therapist) to design a realistic treatment plan, involving reasonably graded goals of exposure and achievement, which can be uniquely tailored to the individual's needs and capabilities. The benefits of home assessment of agoraphobia are summarised in Box 4.3.

Diagnosis

Agoraphobia is so commonly associated with panic attacks that the principal diagnostic criteria used (ICD-10 and DSM-IV) differentiate between 'agoraphobia *with* panic attacks' and 'agoraphobia *without* panic attacks'. Diagnosis is usually straightforward and is based on a history of anxiety or panic attacks in public places resulting in avoidance of such situations (*see* Appendix 4A for diagnostic criteria).

Box 4.3   The benefits of home assessment of agoraphobia

- may be the *only* way of assessing such patients
- ability to observe the patient within their home environment
- permits assessment of degree to which patient's lifestyle is restricted
- allows judgements to be made about how well the patient is coping
- enables additional information to be gleaned from relatives
- may enhance the doctor–patient relationship
- allows judgements to be made concerning the degree to which family members might be reinforcing the avoidant behaviour
- allows identification of family members who may act as 'therapy facilitators'
- enables the design of a realistic treatment plan uniquely tailored to the individual

---

The general rubric for the ICD-10 diagnostic criteria for agoraphobia describes:

a fairly well-defined cluster of phobias embracing fears of leaving home, entering shops, crowds and public places, or travelling alone in trains, buses or planes. Panic disorder is a frequent feature of both present and past episodes. Depressive and obsessional symptoms and social phobias are also commonly present as subsidiary features. Avoidance of the phobic situation is often prominant, and some agoraphobics experience little anxiety because they are able to avoid the phobic situations.

Treatment of agoraphobia

Medical management

The role of the GP in the treatment of agoraphobia is primarily one of assessment, both of the condition itself and of associated complications, such as depression and alcohol abuse. The treatment of depression is considered elsewhere (*see* Wilkinson, Moore and Moore, 1999). In the current text the main focus of attention is the treatment of the core features of agoraphobia.

Drugs play a limited role in the management of agoraphobia, the most robust treatment strategy being behavioural therapy. However, where there is severe and disabling anxiety, which prevents the patient successfully engaging in conventional approaches, then medication has a valuable role to play in reducing anxiety symptoms; this in turn allows the patient to pursue the inevitable course of behavioural therapy or 'cure by exposure'.

Pharmacotherapy

There are two principal classes of drugs which can be used in agoraphobia, namely SSRIs and benzodiazepines. SSRIs are used for long-term therapy of panic associated with agoraphobia, whereas benzodiazepines may be used as a short-term treatment.

SSRIs are helpful only when administered consistently over a sustained period; they should ideally be continued for at least 3 months following remission of symptoms in order to avoid relapse on withdrawal of medication. *They are particularly effective in cases of agoraphobia complicated by panic attacks.* As discussed in Chapter 5, those SSRIs specifically licenced for the treatment of panic attacks are also indicated in the treatment of agoraphobia. Appropriately licenced drugs are citalopram and paroxetine, and these are listed in Box 4.4.

Benzodiazepines should only be used with caution in treating agoraphobia, on account of their tendency to produce dependence. Ideally they should only be prescribed a few tablets at a time, with instructions to use them only if it is unavoidable. A long-acting benzodiazepine is recommended, such as diazepam 2–5 mg prn up to three times daily (just before leaving the house, for example) and for no more than a few days at a time. This regimen should be used only as

---

Box 4.4 Drugs used in the treatment of agoraphobia with panic attacks

Citalopram: initially 10 mg daily, rising fortnightly to 20–30 mg daily (max. 60 mg)

Paroxetine: initially 10 mg daily, rising fortnightly to 20–40 mg daily (max. 50 mg)

Diazepam: 2 mg prn up to TDS before entering feared situation; review every few days. NB as part of an overall management plan involving graded exposure

part of an overall management plan involving graded exposure therapy (usually with a community psychiatric nurse).

Psychological treatment of agoraphobia

As stated above, the mainstay of treatment for agoraphobia is psychological. This comprises both a behavioural and cognitive approach, which is usually carried out by a mental health nurse (community psychiatric nurse or community mental health nurse). In order to avoid repetition, the psychological management of agoraphobia is discussed, together with the psychological management of other phobias, towards the end of this chapter.

Simple phobias

Phobic states comprise intense dread of certain objects or specific situations which would not normally have that effect. Anxiety tends to spread from a specified situation or object to a wider range of circumstances and becomes indistinguishable from other anxiety states. Classically, the main feature of this disorder is a persistent fear of a specific object or situation, or of humiliation or embarrassment in certain social situations. This fear is out of proportion to the demands of the situation and cannot be explained or reasoned away; it is also beyond voluntary control and leads to avoidance of the feared situation.

Simple phobias are sometimes called specific phobias (*see* Box 4.5). The most common in the general population involve animals, particularly dogs, snakes, insects and mice. Other simple phobias involve blood,

---

Box 4.5 Simple phobias

- Women outnumber men for animal phobias, otherwise sex incidence is equal
- Persistent irrational fear of, and compelling desire to avoid, an object or a situation other than being alone in public places away from home (agoraphobia) or of embarrassment in certain social settings (social phobia)
- Relative absence of other psychiatric symptoms
- Tends to pursue continuous course

tissue injury, closed spaces (claustrophobia), heights (acrophobia) and air travel.

Typically this particular type of phobic disorder is chronic and the associated impairment is severe. Moreover, illness phobia is associated with excessive medical consultations and often unnecessary physical investigations, which themselves tend to feed the phobia rather than assuage it. Box 4.6 provides general information concerning this rare but important condition.

Box 4.6 Features of illness phobia

- **Epidemiology**
  - 15% of such phobic patients consult a psychiatrist
  - occurs equally in both sexes
  - a persistent intense fear of illness focused on specific disorders such as cancer, heart disease, mental illness or an intense fear of death and dying
  - chronic ruminations but no apparent attempts at resistance
  - previous illness in relative or individual may act as precipitant
  - may have other mental disorder (e.g. depression) and illness phobia abates as this is treated

- **Predisposing and associated factors**
  - passive, anxious and dependent pre-morbid personalities
  - stable families
  - similar to general population in education and social class
  - often precipitated by a major life event
  - history of childhood fears and enuresis
  - higher incidence of sexual problems in female group compared with control population

- **Course and prognosis**
  - fluctuating course
  - may persist for many years when established

Animal phobias

Animal phobias are rarely seen in general practice, or indeed in psychiatry. This probably reflects a predominantly urban culture in which daily contact with animals is not required, a fact which permits people with animal phobia to effectively avoid the feared stimulus without significantly affecting their lifestyle or health. Animal phobia nearly always begins in childhood and if severe may come to the attention of health professionals. Effective trreatment, as described later in this chapter, involves graded exposure therapy, which is usually carried out either by a child psychologist or an appropriately trained nurse specialist.

Other simple phobias

These are relatively rare, but some forms of specific phobia are particularly important in the health setting. These include needle, blood and injury phobias, which tend to arise in childhood or adolescence, and have important implications where physical treatment is required (ranging from dentistry to diabetes). Again, treatment is primarily psychological, although in the acute setting drug sedation may be indicated.

Fears of heights, driving, closed spaces and air travel appear to begin most frequently in adulthood, but rarely concern medical personnel except where routine avoidance of these triggers is unavoidable.

Social phobia

Here the focus of anxiety is upon social situations (rather than being confined, in crowds or being alone). The main experience is of a persistent fear of one or more social situations in which the patient is, or believes him/herself to be, under scrutiny by others and fears that he or she will do something humiliating or embarrassing (see Box 4.7).

Patients may fear social gatherings where they are expected to talk to others, and may be particularly worried about becoming conspicuous, perhaps by blushing or becoming unable to speak or even vomiting. Parties, meals with other people and business meetings are amongst the most stressful situations. Other examples include fears of drinking with

---

> **Box 4.7**   General points regarding social phobia
>
> - 60% women
> - usually develops after puberty and peaks in late teens.
> - persistent irrational fear of, and compelling desire to avoid, situations in which the individual may be exposed to the scrutiny of others
> - the fear that individual may behave in a manner (blushing, shaking, vomiting) that will be humiliating or embarrassing
> - probably represents the prominent symptomatic manifestation of a wide variety of psychological disorders

others, using a public toilet or even signing documents or cheques in front of other people.

In common with most forms of anxiety, the feared situation becomes anticipated and the cycle of fear worsens, leading to avoidance. Sufferers from social phobias, however, may develop strategies to avoid some difficulties which may prevent more serious social withdrawal. For example, someone may claim not to drink tea or coffee when at meetings or 'forget' reading glasses in order to avoid signing documents under the scrutiny of others.

Social phobia and natural shyness

The news media has been quick to comment on the medical management of what is considered to be natural 'shyness'; such views reflect an incomplete understanding of social phobia as a disorder. The present text does not propose to discuss either the philosophical basis or the ethical implications of 'medicating personality'. Suffice it to say that social phobia can be seen as an extreme form of what may pass for normal shyness; however, in social phobia the patient experiences anxiety symptoms which are so severe that social interaction is actually *avoided*, or endured only with significant *distress*.

Treatment of social phobia

This kind of anxiety has been shown to respond to treatment with the SSRI paroxetine, in a dose of 20–40 mg daily; ideally this should be given for at least 6 months, and in combination with a cognitive-behaviour approach in order to reduce the risk of relapse.

Psychological treatment of phobias

Behavioural therapy and anxiety management are potent tools in the treatment of anxiety-related disorders, and need not be carried out by a GP or psychiatrist. Usually such therapy is the premise of a trained community mental health nurse (previously community psychiatric nurse); exposure therapy is ideally executed in and around the patient's own home, and when suitably advanced may allow the individual to attend an anxiety-management group in the locality (typically in a community mental health resource centre – day hospital).

As with CBT for all the anxiety-related disorders, the principal aim of therapy is to approach the feared object or situation and learn how to respond to it in more adaptive ways. This is achieved by graded exposure and systematic desensitisation. If the tendency to escape, avoid or withdraw from phobic situations is reversed, the patient has the opportunity to learn that in reality the situation is not dangerous. Treatment therefore requires patients to repeatedly make contact with things they fear, remaining in contact with them until the fear starts to subside. Exposure thus breaks the vicious circle that maintain symptoms, and facilitates new learning. By facing the feared objects, patients re-learn how to deal with them effectively.

Treatment rationale

It is important to begin treatment by explaining the model in Figure 4.1, incorporating the patient's individual symptoms to illustrate how vicious circles maintain their symptoms. The principle of exposure and prevention of avoidance follows quite clearly from the model. It should be explained to patients that although they will be expected to come into contact with the things they fear, this will be done in a gradual fashion and not until they feel relatively confident in applying the anxiety-reducing stategies taught to them.

I Behavioural aspects

Exposure and systematic desensitisation

The phobic individual imagines a series of increasingly frightening scenes whilst in a state of deep relaxation. The identification of the range of feared situations and objects is facilitated by the use of a hierarchy or 'fear ladder' (*see* Figure 3.5). Further details on how to construct a hierarchy and proceed with graded exposure are given in Chapter 3.

An example of a hierarchy for fear of heights is shown in Table 4.1. Try to incorporate a wide range of feared situations and include modulating factors, e.g. the presence of trusted others, proximity to

Table 4.1 Hierarchy for fear of heights

	Rating scale (0–100)
1 Look over bannisters on upstairs landing	5
2 Look through closed first-floor window	7
3 Lean out of first-floor window	10
4 As above at friend's house, with second-floor window	10–20
5 Look down from plate glass window in an office, work up to the sixth floor	30–40
6 Look down from top of 'down-going' escalator	35
7 Use step ladder to change light bulb in centre of room	40
8 Walk across bridge over river, close to handrail	50
9 Drive over suspension bridge	60
10 Church tower: walk up and onto roof	70
11 Walk along cliff path	80
12 Drive along mountain roads, e.g. in North Wales	90
13 Eat a meal in the Post Office Tower	100

Some ways of devising a variety of tasks relevant to this hierarchy:

• working on stairs and windows in increasingly unfamiliar places

• doing each task first with someone, then alone

• watching films or looking at pictures of rock climbing, window cleaners, trapeze artists, aeroplane flights, ski-jumping, etc.

• practising looking down, allowing time for the eyes to become adjusted, e.g. by focusing on items at ever-increasing distances.

Adapted from Hawton *et al.* (1992).

feared object, etc. As well as exposure to images and thoughts relating to the feared object, it is important to undertake exposure *in vivo*, that is, in real-life phobic situations.

Initiating exposure can be facilitated by the therapist acting as a 'model', demonstrating how to approach the phobic object whilst being observed by the patient. Modelling has been found to be most effective when the model exhibits, and overcomes, anxiety; observing such a 'coping model' enhances the patient's own coping skills as it shows them what works in that situation and how to do it.

Anxiety-management techniques

Various anxiety-management strategies are learnt by the patient to enable them to remain in contact with their feared stimulus until anxiety levels begin to fall. Effective strategies have been discussed elsewhere (*see* Chapters 3 and 9) and comprise progressive muscular relaxation, breathing retraining, role-playing, rehearsal and modelling. Cognitive strategies such as mental distraction, identifying thoughts and finding alternatives are also useful in reducing anxiety during exposure and simultaneously help to educate the patient and adapt their thought processes.

Self-monitoring

The patient should be encouraged to keep records of their progress in using the hierarchy to facilitate exposure. This enables them to monitor their own anxiety levels, reminds them to continue with tasks between sessions and enhances their self-esteem when progress is evident. In addition, it forces them to attend to their successful attempts to face their fears, rather than perpetuating the natural negative bias, which selectively recalls failures and negative events and ignores positive outcomes. Written records provide important information at times of relapse or setbacks. Different types of recording sheet are provided in Appendix 2.

Group treatment

Similarities between phobics make them suitable for treatment in groups. Members of a group are able to share ideas about coping and provide each other with support and encouragement. Social phobics benefit from understanding they are not alone in their fears and group exposure can be planned, or social events within the group can be attempted, knowing the other members will be sympathetic to their social difficulties. Group exposure for agoraphobics is usually planned around a joint expedition to a local town or shopping area, where members can work on their tasks singly or in pairs depending upon their needs and level of progress.

Family/spouse involvement

Enrolling the help of a spouse or friend to act as co-therapist enables the patient to continue with exposure exercises between therapy sessions. This will also, hopefully, teach friends and family members how they can appropriately help the patient and prevent inadvertant reinforcement of avoidance or dependence behaviour. This is particularly important in the treatment of agoraphobics; it has been posited that, by being overly solicitous and supportive, the spouse or family members may have unwittingly conspired to perpetuate the agoraphobia. Marital and sexual difficulties may emerge as treatment progresses and as the patient becomes less dependent, raising the possibility that the phobic behaviour was serving some useful function within the relationship. Couple therapy or family therapy may be required to help the family system adjust to the changes brought about by the patient's recovery.

2 Cognitive aspects

Identifying anxious thoughts

Social phobia has obvious cognitive components, e.g. thoughts about being negatively evaluated, criticised or rejected. The cognitive aspects of agoraphobia are more likely to focus on the possibility of collapsing or losing control. A wide variety of simple phobias are maintained by thoughts of harm arising from proximity to the feared stimulus. The cognitive content of individuals' thoughts are often idiosyncratic. They can usually be identified by asking 'When you are feeling anxious, what is in your mind?' or 'What is the worst that could happen?'. The content of patients' anxious or catastrophic thoughts then become the focus of therapy, as covered in other chapters.

Modifying anxious thoughts

Patients' fearful thoughts become the target of appropriate exposure exercises and 'behavioural tests'. With repeated practice in approaching those situations or objects they most fear, their cognitions about the dangerousness of their proximity to the stimulus and the threat posed to them by not fleeing will change. The aim of applying cognitive techniques alongside behavioural exposure is to facilitate the adaptation of their anxious thoughts via the process of cognitive reappraisal; in CBT, patients learn through their own experiences, during exposure, that their anxious thoughts do not reflect reality. For example, a woman with agoraphobia who becomes able to walk to the local shops on her own without disastrous consequences, reappraises the way she interprets the situation. She is now able to see her anxious thoughts as irrational and catastrophic; she neither collapsed nor made a show of herself by losing control. In addition, cognitions relating to self-esteem are also altered by patients' new perceptions of themselves as being able to cope with adverse circumstances.

Cognitive therapists may also ask the individual to search for evidence that firstly, confirms their anxious thought and then look for evidence to disconfirm that same thought. So, the thought 'If I get near to a dog, it will bite me', may be confirmed by the fact that once, when they were a child, they were bitten by a dog. However, it can be disconfirmed numerous times once they begin to approach dogs and stop avoiding them. A suitable recording sheet is shown in Figure 4.2.

Monitoring cognitive change

As with cognitive techniques in treating panic disorder (see Chapter 5), patients' erroneous interpretations and catastrophic predictions need to be identified and examined. Alternative, and more plausible, explanations are then generated and tested systematically during exposure. For example, social phobics may expect others to be unfriendly, disinterested or critical. However, if they smile at an acquaintance, they may receive a smile in return, and if they ask a question or disclose something about themselves they may end up beginning a conversation. These events thereby disconfirm their original predictions. In this way cognitive procedures enable the patient to assimilate new information gathered during exposure tasks and enhance the alteration in thinking that is necessary for long-term change. Regular monitoring of the ensuing adaptation in patients' cognitions can be facilitated by the use of recording sheets (see Chapter 3, Figures 3.4 and 3.6).

Training techniques specific to social phobia

Social skills training. Anxiety in social phobics is thought to be somewhat related to a lack of appropriate social skills. According to this view, the

Balance sheet for thoughts

My thought: _____

EVIDENCE IN FAVOUR OF MY THOUGHT Note past situations where this thought was true	EVIDENCE AGAINST MY THOUGHTS Be alert for situations which disprove your negative thought

Figure 4.2 Thoughts balance sheet.

individual has not learnt how to behave so that they feel comfortable in social situations; they feel awkward and socially inept, imagining they are being evaluated harshly by their companions. Socially anxious people are rated by others as being low in social skills and their timing and responses in social interaction are impaired. These faults can be corrected during specific training addressing such social skills as: starting a conversation, picking up on cues from the other person, non-verbal communication, etc. Training usually takes place in groups where repeated practice, video-recording and 'feedback' techniques are employed.

Assertiveness training. People with social phobia may also benefit from specific training in how to be assertive in difficult social interactions. Being assertive basically means being able to express your views about some issue in a way that is acceptable to, and understood by, the other person. Assertiveness maintains the balance between passive behaviour on the one hand, and aggressive responses on the other. Therapists may incorporate role-play, modelling and role-reversal techniques in training the individual in assertion skills. The patient is encouraged to role-play a particular social interaction or event which they avoid, before observing the therapist modelling the correct assertiveness skills and then switching roles to enable them to become familiar with the skills required for that situation. Common themes in assertiveness training involve: taking faulty goods back to a shop, someone 'jumping the queue' ahead of you, refusing to do a favour and asking someone for a favour.

Preventing relapse

Clearly, relapse will be reduced by the patient having a thorough working knowledge of the behavioural and cognitive procedures employed in therapy. Throughout therapy sesssions increasing emphasis should be given to the patient devising their own exposure tasks and explaining their cognitive changes to the therapist. However, minor set-backs are likely, particularly at times of increased stress. At these times it is useful to have an individualised sheet with instructions to the patient regarding how to continue with their own treatment. This sheet is ideally compiled by the patient towards the end of therapy, in collaboration with the therapist, who can direct them to the techniques they have learned which have been effective for them. Box 4.8 gives an example of a set-back sheet.

Box 4.8 Patient's individualised sheet to prevent relapse

My setback sheet (or what to do if things slip back)

1 Don't shy away from doing things that are difficult. Do them quickly, before you have time to worry again
2 Remember how many times you had to visit the post office before you felt OK. Now even the shops in town are OK
3 Do the relaxation exercises properly once a month as a reminder. (NB Write this in diary so it doesn't get forgotten)
4 Don't get bogged down in the horror of it all: it's more encouraging to think about the progress I have made before, and what to do next. Write down the steps involved
5 Look back at old record sheets. They show which order I did things before, and how much practice I had to do before it got easier
6 Go into the supermarket alone sometimes. Don't always go with the family, even if it's more convenient to do so
7 Plan to go to all the school concerts next term
8 Breathe slowly when you feel bad
9 Watch out for thinking the worst will happen. It hasn't happened yet!

If things get difficult again:

- Remember setbacks happen to everyone. You can't get through life without having some bad times

- Work out how to practise in steps. Write the steps down, and make sure you tackle them one by one. Write down how you felt each time

- Practise every day. There's no need to run before you can walk

- Don't bottle it up. Talk to the family about what's happening

Appendix 4A

ICD-10 diagnostic criteria for agoraphobia

A There is marked and consistently manifest fear in, or avoidance of, at least two of the following situations:

- crowds

- public places

- travelling alone

- travelling away from home.

B At least two symptoms of anxiety in the feared situation must have been present together, on at least one occasion since the onset of the disorder, and one of the symptoms must have been from items 1–4 below:

- autonomic arousal symptoms

  (1) palpitations or pounding or accelerated heart rate
  (2) sweating
  (3) trembling or shaking
  (4) dry mouth (not due to medication or dehydration)

- symptoms involving chest and abdomen

  (5) difficulty breathing
  (6) feeling of choking
  (7) chest pain or discomfort
  (8) nausea or abdominal distress (e.g. churning in stomach)

- symptoms involving mental state

  (9) feeling dizzy, unsteady, faint or light-headed
  (10) derealisation or depersonalisation
  (11) fear of losing control, 'going crazy' or passing out
  (12) fear of dying

- general symptoms

   (13) hot flushes or cold chills
   (14) numbness or tingling sensations.

C Significant emotional distress is caused by the avoidance of anxiety symptoms, and the individual recognises that these are excessive or unreasonable.

D Symptoms are restricted to, or predominate in, the feared situations or contemplation of them.

Phobic disorders – F40

Adapted from WHO (1996)

Includes agoraphobia, social phobia.

Presenting complaints

- Patients may avoid or restrict activities because of fear.
- They may have difficulty travelling to the doctor's office, going shopping, visiting others.
- Patients sometimes present with physical symptoms (palpitations, shortness of breath, 'asthma'). Questioning will reveal specific fears.

Diagnostic features

Unreasonably strong fear of specific places or events. Patients often **avoid** these situations altogether. Patients may be **unable to leave home** or unable to stay alone because of fear. Commonly feared situations include:

- leaving home
- open spaces
- speaking in public
- crowds or public places
- travelling in buses, cars, trains or planes
- social events.

Differential diagnosis

- If anxiety attacks are prominent see *Panic attacks – F41.0.*

- If low or sad mood is prominent, see *Depression – F32#.*

- Many of the management guidelines given below may also be helpful for specific phobias (e.g. fear of water, fear of heights).

Phobic disorders – F40: management guidelines

Essential information for patient and family

- Phobias can be treated.

- **Avoiding feared situations allows the fear to grow stronger.**

- **Following a set of specific steps can help a person overcome fear.**

Counselling of patient and family

- Encourage the patient to practise **controlled breathing methods** to reduce physical symptoms of fear.

- Ask the patient to make a list of all situations that he/she fears and avoids although other people do not.

- **Discuss ways to challenge these exaggerated fears** (e.g. patient reminds him/herself, 'I am feeling a little anxious because there is a large crowd. The feeling will pass in a few minutes.').

- Plan a **series of steps to enable the patient to confront and get used to** feared situations:

  - identify a small first step towards the feared situation (e.g. take a short walk away from home with a family member)
  - this step should be practised for 1 hour each day until it is no longer frightening
  - if the feared situation still causes anxiety, the patient should practise slow and relaxed breathing, telling him/herself that the panic will pass within 30 minutes. The patient should not leave the feared situation until the fear subsides
  - move on to a slightly more difficult step and repeat the procedure (e.g. spend a longer time away from home)

- take no alcohol or anti-anxiety medicine for at least 4 hours before practising these steps.

- Identify a **friend or family member who will help** in overcoming the fear. Self-help groups can assist in confronting feared situations.

- The patient should avoid using alcohol or benzodiazepine drugs to cope with feared situations.

Medication

- With the use of these counselling methods, many patients will not need medication. However, if depression is also present, antidepressant medication may be helpful (e.g. imipramine 50–150 mg a day).

- For patients with infrequent and limited symptoms, occasional use of anti-anxiety medication (e.g. benzodiazepines) may help. Regular use may lead to dependence, however, and is likely to result in return of symptoms when discontinued.

- For management of performance anxiety (e.g. fear of public speaking) beta-blockers may reduce physical symptoms.

Specialist consultation

Consider consultation if disabling fears (e.g. patient is unable to leave home) persist. Referral for behavioural psychotherapy, if available, may be effective for patients who do not improve.

5
Panic attacks

The term 'panic' derives from Pan, the dwarf-like god of ancient Greek mythology; he would hide in his cave waiting for a human to pass by, only to jump out screaming at the unsuspecting traveller. The unmistakable response provoked justly earned the epithet Pan-ic, traditionally characterised as being 'scared to death'.

Panic *disorder* essentially comprises recurrent and unpredictable attacks of intense anxiety. Interestingly, and in contrast to other anxiety disorders, panic attacks as a discrete nosological entity have only gained international recognition quite recently; in the 1960's panic attacks were still generally seen only as symptoms of other disorders such as generalised anxiety, depression or agoraphobia. The acceptance of panic disorder as a discrete diagnostic category was recognised by its inclusion in the third edition of the Diagnostic and Statistical Manual of Diseases (DSM-III) in 1980, and it has subsequently been included in ICD-10 in 1992.

Epidemiology

Unfortunately the epidemiology of panic disorder remains poorly understood, largely reflecting the differences in diagnostic tools used to measure 'caseness'. In a review of existing estimates, Sartorius (1996) give a prevalence of around 1% of the population suffering from panic disorder at any time. However, as it is usually treatable (i.e. the illness does not equate with a lifetime diagnosis) it is likely that the number of people who have *ever* had panic attacks is far greater, and the lifetime risk may be in the order of 10%.

The onset of panic disorder usually arises in the 20s; it is uncommon under the age of 15, and new cases after the age of 40 are rare. The sex distribution of 'pure' panic disorder (i.e. panic independent of other anxiety syndromes) is roughly equal between males and females;

however, panic associated with agoraphobia is three times more common in women than in men.

Natural history

Untreated, the illness appears to run one of two courses: either the panic becomes associated with specific situations (e.g. crowded places) leading to avoidance behaviour, in which case it is subsumed under a different diagnostic category such as phobic anxiety (in particular agoraphobia); or the disorder leads to a depressive illness, which may be seen as resulting from the suffering associated with recurrent panic. Rarely, panic disorder runs a chronic course, tending to abate as the individual gets older.

Box 5.1 Case example 1

Mr D, a 22-year-old student, experienced his first panic attack 14 months previously when on a university geological field trip. This involved a number of students sleeping on the wooden floor of an outbuilding; when getting ready to go to sleep on the first night his heart began pounding and he suddenly became terrified, thinking he was going to die. He was breathless, sweating and shaking all over, and had to be reassured repeatedly by the trip organiser, until the symptoms abated over the next few minutes. His next attack was 2 weeks later, and since that time he had experienced similar attacks most weeks without warning and in various settings. He had subsequently read a self-help book on panic attacks and had learned to control the intensity and duration of episodes, but he eventually requested specialist referral as he wanted to be completely free from the distressing attacks.

Approximately one-third of panic attacks occur in public places, one-third at home and one-quarter whilst driving or being driven in a car. A period of stress usually precedes the first panic, and in many cases there is an identifiable precipitant (e.g. work stress, bereavement, personal conflicts). After the initial panic, medical assurance that there is no physical illness gives short-lived relief; the mysterious and distressing nature of the attacks remains unexplained and may give rise to further anxiety. Although ICD-10 requires that a discrete diagnosis of panic disorder should only be made if the attacks are 'not consistently associated with a situation or object', a clinical description of panic attacks should make mention of panic which *is* associated with specific situations. Rachman and de Silva (1996) provide detailed accounts of the various types of panic attack in their book *Panic Disorder: the facts.*

- **Unexpected panic.** This represents the 'pure' form of panic disorder as defined by ICD-10. Attacks occur 'out of the blue' and with no obvious trigger or threat to explain them.

- **Situational panic.** Most panic attacks occur in response to a perceived threat; this may be imagined or exaggerated in the mind of the individual, and subsequent panics are provoked by situations similar to the precipitating event.

- **Anticipatory panic.** This follows from situational panic; attacks occur even at the prospect of encountering the feared situation.

- **Nocturnal panic.** Nocturnal panic is reported in about one-quarter of people suffering with panic attacks, and typically occurs during the early hours of sleep. These attacks tend to be more severe than those occurring in the day, and frequently last for 25 minutes or more.

- **Relaxation-induced panic.** These attacks appear to arise from a fear of losing control, which may be associated with progressive muscular relaxation techniques (where indicated, relaxation based on mental imagery should be used).

- **Drug-induced panic.** Illicit recreational drug use, in particular cannabis, frequently gives rise to panic attacks in first-time users. This usually deters further use of the drug, but occasionally leads to subsequent panic attacks in the absence of the drug.

Cued and uncued panic

A widely accepted broad classification of panic attacks relates simply to the presence or absence of triggers or 'cues'. Hence, panic attacks associated with situational triggers are termed *cued* panic attacks, and include all of the above categories except for 'unexpected' panic attacks.

Uncued panic attacks must arise in the absence of situational triggers and constitute panic *disorder*.

Box 5.2   Case example 2

A 30-year-old schoolteacher, Mrs C, had her first panic attack on returning home from shopping. She had a number of bags to fetch from the car, which she had left open in the road. It was dusk and just beginning to rain when she suddenly felt extremely tight-chested as if she could not breathe. She caught hold of the front door for support, breathing in and out very rapidly, her mouth dry and her body shaking all over, and terrified that she was going mad. Her son came to the door and, frightened for his mother, immediately called for an ambulance. She was still in a state of extreme panic when the ambulance crew arrived 10 minutes later and in spite of efforts to reassure her it was not until she was lightly sedated in casualty that her symptoms began to resolve. Physical tests were all normal and she was referred to the psychiatric team; during treatment over the next few weeks she improved quickly, and only had four minor panic attacks over the next month, being symptom-free at 6-month follow-up.

Aetiology

As with the other anxiety disorders, the cause of panic attacks is not to be found in any single modality, but is multifactorial. Thus, it appears that those who are both genetically predisposed to panic; and exposed to environmental risk factors, are more likely to develop panic disorder when they experience an initiating or precipitating event. Psychological factors such as loss of control may then contribute to maintaining the illness. These areas will be considered separately.

Genes

The evidence available from twin studies of panic disorder is, as yet, too sparse to yield any conclusive data concerning the heritability of the illness. There is a slightly increased risk of panic disorder in close relatives of probands (subjects with the illness), but it is unclear to what extent this is a result of genetic or environmental factors. Nevertheless, genes have been shown to be important in predisposing individuals to other forms of anxiety disorder, and this seems likely to be the case for panic attacks as well.

Environment

Research has identified a number of environmental risk factors, exposure to which increases the likelihood of an individual developing panic attacks. These include a history of family conflict, lack of parental support and separation anxiety in childhood. Other risk factors are a chronic physical or psychiatric illness in the family, and the abuse of alcohol or drugs in the family. These risk factors are summarised in Box 5.3.

Box 5.3 Risk factors for panic attacks

- history of family conflict
- lack of parental support
- separation anxiety in childhood
- chronic physical or psychiatric illness in the family
- the abuse of alcohol or drugs in the family

Neurobiology

The neurobiological basis of panic shares essential features with the biological substrate of anxiety, which has been considered in Chapter 1. The neurobiology and neuroanatomy relating to fear and anxiety will not therefore be repeated here, but only those concepts thought to relate directly to panic attacks.

Arousal mechanisms

The brain can be conceptualised as having excitatory and inhibitory mechanisms, which normally counterpoise each other in order to maintain a level of arousal and behaviour appropriate to the prevailing stimuli, which may be internal (e.g. dyspnoea, hypotension) or external (e.g. threat of attack). Put simply, the arousal system is subserved by noradrenergic projections from the locus coeruleus, and inhibition by the serotonergic fibres of the brain stem raphe nuclei.

Peri-aqueductal grey matter

Animal studies have shown that stimulation of the **PAG** produces fight or flight responses. Serotonergic fibres inhibit the PAG and attenuate the fear response. Noradrenergic fibres from the locus coeruleus, however, have a stimulating effect on the PAG, thus enhancing the fight or flight response; it is thought that *intermittent* surges of noradrenergic input to the PAG is associated with panic attacks, whereas a *continuous* high input is *not*. Although the current theory is rather crude, the concept of intermittent versus continuous noradrenergic activity appears to be consistent with pharmacological approaches to panic disorder. These ideas are summarised diagrammatically in Figure 5.1.

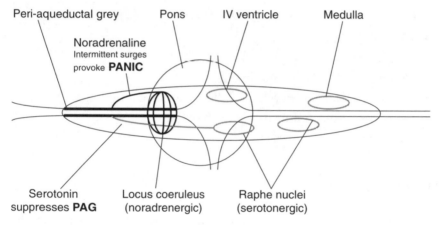

Figure 5.1 Proposed neurobiology of panic.

Panicogens and adrenaline

Laboratory findings have shown that panic attacks can be induced by an intravenous infusion of sodium lactate. This occurs in the majority of subjects who suffer with panic attacks and in a small proportion of normal controls. The fact that lactate is metabolised to carbon dioxide implies that panic may be a 'suffocation response' to an oversensitive 'suffocation alarm', although this theory has yet to be substantiated.

Substances inducing panic are called **panicogens**, and include yohimbine, doxapram and cholecystekinin, as well as cannabis and cocaine.

The systemic form of noradrenaline is **adrenaline**, named after its association with the ad*renal* (by *kidney*) gland, and when produced inappropriately it may cause symptoms of panic. Brainstem arousal, as described above, leads to autonomic discharge, particularly sympathetic, which is associated with a sudden systemic release of adrenaline; this gives rise to an almost instantaneous rise in heart rate and blood pressure normally required for a fight or flight response. However, in the absence of a threat or stimulus no rapid action ensues and the subject is left experiencing the symptoms of sympathetic arousal, which may be misattributed to serious illness.

Subliminal stimuli in an already stressed (and hence *primed*) individual may provoke transient brainstem stimulation with consequent adrenaline release and sympathetic arousal; fear that these arousal sensations may be due to life-threatening illness leads to increased central nervous arousal (by positive biofeedback) and immediately a cycle is created. This cycle may be termed the psychosomatic model of panic and it is shown diagrammatically in Figure 5.2.

Clinical features of panic

In approaching the assessment of panic it is necessary to bear in mind the distinction between the terms *panic attacks* and *panic disorder*. Panic *attacks* are seen in a number of psychiatric disorders, including agoraphobia, generalised anxiety and depression. Panic attacks occurring in isolation comprise panic *disorder*.

In panic disorder, panic attacks are paroxysms of intense fear and dread, which strike suddenly, without warning and for no apparent reason (case examples are given in Boxes 5.1 and 5.2). The symptoms of panic are both physical and psychological. Physical symptoms are predominantly cardiovascular and include palpitations, shortness of breath, sweating and trembling; there may also be a feeling of choking, chest pain, nausea, paraesthesiae, dry mouth and faintness. The psychological symptoms are marked by feelings of intense terror, together with a sense of 'the self not being there' (depersonalisation) or of 'the world not being real' (derealisation); in addition there is often a fear of dying, or of losing control or going mad. Typically, each attack tends to 'burn itself out' after 10 or 20 minutes. The full range of symptoms recorded in ICD-10 is given in the appendix to this chapter (*see* p. 112).

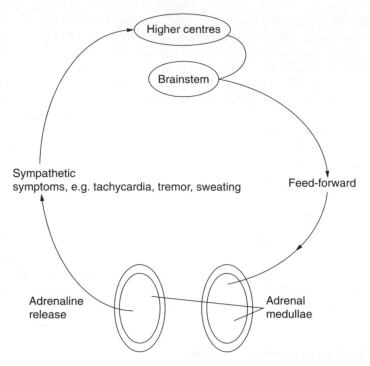

Figure 5.2 The psychosomatic model of panic.

Comorbidity

As discussed above, panic attacks (not panic disorder) may be associated with a number of other psychiatric conditions. Fifty per cent of people with panic disorder have suffered from major depression at some time in their lives; 25% have had social phobia and 25% have had features of obsessive-compulsive disorder; around 20% have had alcohol problems (Rachman and de Silva, 1996). The frequency of these associated conditions is summarised in Box 5.4.

Agoraphobia

Interestingly, there is a lack of meaningful data on the frequency of agoraphobia associated with panic attacks. This is probably due to the fact that when people with panic attacks develop agoraphobia, they may

> **Box 5.4** Psychiatric illness associated with panic attacks
>
> * 40% current depression
> * 50% history of depression
> * 25% history of social phobia
> * 25% history of obsessive-compulsive features
> * 20% history of alcohol problems

cease having panic attacks as long as they avoid the feared situation (e.g. crowded places). Hence, such agoraphobics may not have had a typical panic attack for many years and as a result do not fulfil diagnostic criteria for panic attacks. (The management of agoraphobia is considered in Chapter 4.).

Assessment

Many patients presenting to the family doctor already have an idea that they are suffering from panic attacks, either because they have been diagnosed in casualty or they are familiar with panic attacks through relatives or the media. Hence, routine diagnosis of panic attacks is usually reasonably straightforward. Nevertheless, a careful history of the attacks is always necessary in order to exclude other seizure disorders.

Emergency assessment

It is beyond the scope of this text to describe in detail the acute assessment of a panic attack in the emergency department. In brief, the clinician must be satisfied that the patient is neither in respiratory distress (e.g. as a result of acute asthma, pneumothorax or choking) nor suffering from acute cardiac insufficiency (e.g. myocardial infarction). In addition illicit drugs, flashbacks and phaeochromocytoma should also be considered; routine investigations include blood gases, biochemistry, electrocardiogram and chest X-ray. Management then involves calming the patient by means of constant reassurance, and if necessary with light sedation (e.g. oral or intravenous diazepam). Where the patient is clearly over-breathing then re-breathing into a paper bag is often effective in reducing symptoms.

Routine assessment

Panic attacks should not, however, be diagnosed purely by exclusion of physical cause in the acute episode, for this reason it is important that patients seen in the emergency department are referred for subsequent assessment (*see* Box 5.5).

As a general rule, the more chronic the disorder the longer it takes to treat. Moreover, the timing, onset and features of each attack may give

---

Box 5.5 Routine assessment of panic attacks

- **Nature of attacks**
  - when did the attacks start?
  - does anything provoke them?
  - do they arise 'out of the blue'?
  - can you tell if and when you may have an attack?
  - how long do they last?
  - what are the exact symptoms?
  - what is going through your mind at the time?
  - what do you think the attacks are due to?

- **Other causes**
  - do you use illicit drugs? (if so, elaborate)
  - does anyone in your family have similar attacks?
  - do you or family members have asthma?
  - do you or family members have epilepsy?

- **Complications**
  - how have you been coping with the attacks?
  - how have the attacks affected your life?
    e.g.   (i) relationships
           (ii) going out
           (iii) work

- **Comorbidity**
  - do you feel anxious all the time?
  - do you feel depressed? (if so, biological features and *suicidality*?)
  - do you find youself checking or cleaning unnecessarily?
  - how much alcohol do you use? (elaborate if necessary)

---

clues as to what the sufferer fears is wrong with them, either at the time of, or between, attacks. It is therefore important to elicit the precise nature of the attacks in order to understand what they mean to the individual; some subjects acknowledge that they are well between attacks but may think they are dying of a 'heart attack' during attacks; others may believe they are suffering from a physical condition, such as epilepsy or brain tumour, which causes the episodes of panic. This has implications for management because the greater the degree of insight, the more responsive the subject tends to be to treatment.

Diagnosis

The diagnosis of panic attacks follows from assessment as outlined above; the diagnosis of panic *disorder* specifically, depends upon fulfilling the accepted diagnostic criteria. The ICD-10 and DSM-IV diagnostic criteria for panic disorder are given in the Appendix to this chapter.

Differential diagnosis

There are a number of serious conditions that can give rise to the symptoms seen in panic attacks, indeed, it is the mimicry of certain life-threatening illnesses seen in panic attacks which contributes to the intense fear characteristic of such episodes. The immediately life-threatening conditions, such as acute asthma, will have usually been ruled out by the time the patient presents for routine assessment. Nevertheless, at follow-up the clinician should be aware of other conditions which may mimic panic, and these are summarised in Box 5.6.

Hyperventilation syndrome

Hyperventilation syndrome has features in common with the somatic component of panic, but lacks the characteristic psychological symptoms of intense dread and fear of dying, however, there may be subjective anxiety. The main symptoms are: light-headedness or faintness, breath-lessness and palpitations, sweating, fatigue and stiffness, dry mouth with aerophagy, and globus hystericus and chronic malaise. The physiological mechanisms in hyperventilation syndrome are outlined in Box 5.7.

Treatment is by reassurance and getting patients to recognise and

---

Box 5.6 Differential diagnosis of panic attacks

- respiratory distress
- cardiac disease
- **hyperventilation syndrome**
- phaeocromocytoma
- hyperthyroidism
- drug intoxication (cocaine or cannabis)
- alcohol – pathological intoxication
- flashbacks related to stimulant abuse
- flashbacks related to PTSD
- epilepsy

Box 5.7 Physiological mechanisms in hyperventilation

- physiological effects of reduced PCO_2
- vasoconstriction of cerebral arteries
- reduced availability of oxygen in oxyhaemoglobin
- increased irritability of autonomic, sensory and motor nervous system
- bronchial constriction and tachycardia
- exaggerated sinus rhythm

---

control their rate and depth of breathing, or by asking them to re-breathe into a paper bag held over the nose and mouth until symptoms subside (dangerous for patients with cardiorespiratory problems).

Complications of panic disorder

Panic attacks are associated with considerable comorbidity and they frequently lead to marked decline in psychosocial functioning. Relationships may suffer and jobs be lost or left as the individual descends into a spiral of inability to predict routines, self-reproach and a feeling of helplessness and personal weakness. Such patients (up to 60%) often become clinically depressed. It is therefore extemely important to make specific enquiry about depressive symptoms when assessing panic attacks.

Treatment of panic disorder

As emphasised earlier in this chapter, panic attacks may occur either alone or in the context of another anxiety disorder (e.g. agoraphobia). Where the attacks occur in association with another disorder, this may require additional treatment; in practice, however, there is a great deal of overlap both in terms of symptoms and treatment of anxiety disorders. For the purposes of this section the treatment of panic disorder itself is considered.

Pharmacotherapy

The most important element in treating panic attacks centres on explanation and reassurance. These vital elements of treatment will be discussed in the section on psychological management, but they should not be overlooked when prescribing drugs. Many people with panic attacks respond to explanation and reassurance alone, and it is usually only those with severe and enduring attacks who require medication. Even in these cases, medication alone is unlikely to confer lasting benefit in the absence of some kind of explanation of the disorder.

Drugs to use

In deciding which drug to use in panic disorder, in is useful to conceptualise the disorder in terms of the underlying *tendency* to panic (i.e. the disorder) on the one hand, and the actual panic *attacks* on the other hand. The underlying disorder tends to respond to treatment with SSRIs, whilst discrete panic attacks tend to respond to benzodiazepines. Recent work suggests that abecarnil (a partial benzodiazepine receptor agonist) may be effective in treating the disorder, but the results of randomised, controlled trials are awaited.

Serotonergic agents (SSRIs)

There is some evidence that panic disorder may respond to any SSRI, and efficacy appears to be related to serotonergic potency. For this reason, markedly serotonergic tricyclic antidepressants have been used successfully, in particular imipramine. However, in view of their adverse effects and toxicity, tricyclic antidepressants should be used only in those cases of panic disorder which are unresponsive to SSRIs or where there has previously been a good response to a tricyclic.

Although there is some evidence that any SSRI may be effective in treating panic disorder, only two are currently licensed for this purpose, namely paroxetine and citalopram. Higher doses are needed for the effective treatment of panic disorder than for the treatment of anxiety or depression. It is advisable to continue therapy for 6 months, or for at least 3 months following the remission of symptoms. The SSRI should then be withdrawn over a period of a few weeks to avoid any discontinuation syndrome. The recommended dosing schedules are given in Box 5.8.

Box 5.8 Drug treatment of panic disorder

For the underlying disorder:

either

- citalopram 10 mg daily, increased by 10 mg weekly to a maintenance dose of 20–30 mg daily (max. 60 mg OD) continued for 3 months after remission

or

- paroxetine 10 mg daily, increased by 10 mg weekly to a maintenance dose of 40 mg daily (max. 50 mg OD) continued for 3 months after remission

For panic attacks, if severe:

- alprazolam 250–500 µg prn up to a maximum of 3 mg daily, short-term use. Alternatively, 250–500 µg TDS, reducing over 2–4 weeks

For refractory cases:

- imipramine 75 mg daily in divided doses, increased gradually (against side-effects) to a maintenance dose of 150–200 mg. Not advised in cardiac impaired patients or if suicide risk

- may require specialist referral

NB Early panic disorder usually responds to adequate explanation and reassurance

GABA-ergic agents (benzodiazepines)

The role of benzodiazepines in the treatment of generalised anxiety has already been considered (Chapter 3). The issues of dependence and abuse will not be considered further in the present section, except to comment that panic attacks respond better to the more potent and short-acting benzodiazepines, which tend to be more addictive than longer acting ones. The benzodiazepine which has received most attention in relation to panic is alprazolam, a potent drug with a short half-life. It is useful in the acute treatment of panic attacks and, if taken at the onset of an attack, may ameliorate or even abort the episode. Hence, alprazolam may be administered as required (prn) or on a regular, but reducing, schedule (see Box 5.8). However, rebound worsening of panic attacks has been reported following discontinuation, and for this reason it should not be prescribed as a monotherapy, but in conjunction with an SSRI, and then only for a limited period.

Combined drug therapy

For moderate-to-severe panic disorder it is advisable to prescribe an SSRI at a high maintenance dose for at least 6 months (see Box 5.8). The patient may not derive therapeutic benefit from the SSRI for some weeks, while the dose is titrated upwards. During this period acute relief from panic attacks may be achieved by prescribing prn alprazolam for a limited period, usually 2–4 weeks.

Psychological treatment

Initially the treatment for panic attacks mirrored that for agoraphobia, as most people who suffered panic also tended to fear and avoid such things as public transport, busy places and driving, and were thus diagnosed as agoraphobics. The treatment of choice for agoraphobia is the combined behavioural techniques of **systematic desensitisation** and **exposure** *in vivo*. These behaviour-management techniques have been outlined in Chapters 3 and 4 relating to generalised anxiety and phobias. In both these treatments, the individual is gradually and systematically exposed to the feared objects; in systematic desensitisation, the exposure takes place in imagined rehearsals during relaxation, whereas *in vivo* exposure takes place in real-life situations.

In addition to behavioural approaches, therapists have begun to focus attention on the **cognitive component** in panic and the role that the patient's thoughts, beliefs and expectations have on the aetiology and maintenance of their symptoms. CBT uses a combination of these approaches and has become the mainstay of psychological treatment for panic disorders. The patient's cognitions relating to their fears and associated symptoms are elicited and the therapist aids in the modification and 'testing out' of harmful or erroneous cognitions, thus affecting both their behaviour and thoughts.

Cognitive model of panic

Clark's cognitive model of panic (1986) states that individuals experience panic attacks because they tend to interpret a range of bodily sensations in a catastrophic fashion. They misinterpret these sensations as indicative of an immediately impending mental or physical disaster, such as a heart attack, collapse or insanity. The suggested sequence of events in a panic attack is shown in Figure 5.3.

A wide range of stimuli can provoke attacks, being external (e.g. a situation in which the individual has previously experienced a panic attack) or more often internal (thoughts, images or bodily sensations). If these stimuli are perceived as threatening, a state of apprehension develops, inducing sympathetic arousal and the generation of physio-

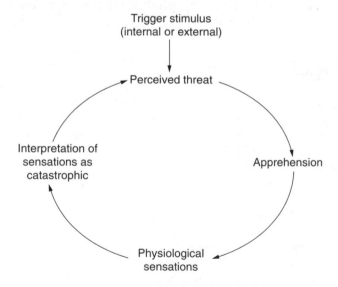

Figure 5.3 The cognitive model of panic (from Clark, 1986).

logical sensations associated with anxiety. If the individual catastrophises about the cause and possible disastrous outcome relating to these symptoms, a further increase in apprehension occurs, producing heightened awareness of increasing sensations, and so on, in a vicious circle that culminates in an attack.

Once an individual has developed a tendency to catastrophically interpret physiological sensations, they will become **hypervigilant**, repeatedly scanning their body for unusual sensations and attaching great meaning to minor symptoms usually ignored. This tends to maintain a panic disorder subsequent to the initial attack. In addition, they **avoid** certain activities or situations, which they believe precipitated the feared sensations, thus maintaining their negative interpretations regarding the disastrous consequences. For example, a patient who is preoccupied with the idea that he is suffering from cardiac disease avoided exercise or sex for fear that it would bring on palpitations. He thus believed that avoiding these activities prevented a heart attack, but his avoidance actually served to reinforce his misinterpretation. By avoiding activity, he was unable to 'test out' the erroneous belief, missing an opportunity to learn that the symptoms he was experiencing were innocuous. He took the reduction in symptoms following avoidance as further evidence that he would have had a heart attack if he had not taken these precautions.

Some panic attacks appear to 'come out of the blue', without identifiable triggers (termed 'pure' panic disorder, without associated anxiety). The bodily sensations misinterpreted here are usually caused, not by heightened anxiety, but by a different emotional state (such as anger, excitement) or by some innocuous event such as suddenly arising from a sitting position (postural hypotension causing dizziness and palpitations) or exercise (breathlessness, palpitations). The patients fail to distinguish between the benign triggering sensations and the subsequent attack, therefore perceiving it as coming 'out of the blue'. Patients often take the absence of obvious triggers as evidence that the attacks are due to some serious physical disorder, therefore helping them identify the antecedents of a spontaneous attack is useful in challenging their catastrophic interpretations.

Description of cognitive-behaviour treatment

Cognitive-behaviour therapy (CBT) aims to reduce panic attacks by teaching patients how to identify, evaluate, control and modify their negative catastrophic thoughts and associated behaviours. Both cognitive and behavioural tehniques are employed; patients are guided towards more appropriate interpretations of their experiences (cognitive component) and are taught how to reduce the intensity and frequency of their disturbing bodily sensations (behavioural component). When choosing specific procedures to use with a particular patient, the therapist is guided by the assessment interview and the hypotheses they developed regarding the main cognitive and behavioural processes maintaining the patient's attacks.

Rationale and education

Early in treatment it is useful to provide patients with written information regarding the nature of anxiety and panic, including the symptoms and their relationship to adrenaline ('the fight or flight' hormone), their possible biological origin and function, reassurring the patients that the associated autonomic changes are not detrimental to their physical health or to their mental sanity. This information is tailored to the particular needs of each patient.

As with CBT treatments for all manner of psychological disorders, the initial objective is to present the rationale underlying the treatment to the patient, ensuring they have a good understanding of the model on which intervention is based. It is helpful to use a simplified version of the model in Figure 5.3 to explain the process, inserting details pertinent to the patient's situation. An example is given in Figure 5.4.

It is important to help the patient identify their specific fears, apprehensions and negative thoughts, as well as their symptoms and possible triggers for attacks. It may take some time before they become familiar with identifying their particular thoughts and catastrophic interpretations for their symptoms. This can be facilitated by the use of panic diaries – *see* Figures 5.5 and 5.6.

It is explained to the patient that treatment consists of them learning certain strategies to break this vicious circle. Modifying their cata-strophic interpretations (the meaning of their bodily sensations) to more realistic ones will break the vicious circle by reducing apprehension, thereby giving rise to fewer sensations. Learning relaxation skills, controlling their breathing and gaining a greater understanding of their symptoms will result in a reduction in the severity and intensity of the bodily sensations. This breaks the circle as gaining control over their bodily sensations reduces the opportunity for making catastrophic interpretations.

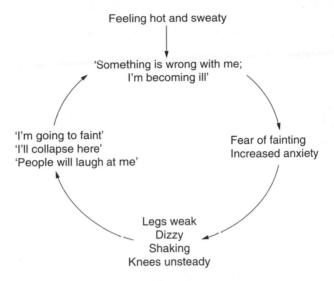

Figure 5.4 Using the cognitive model of panic with a specific example (from Rachman and de Silva, 1996).

Cognitive elements of treatment

Identifying negative thoughts. In order to help the patient in modifying their maladaptive cognitions, they first need to identify them. This is often facilitated by getting patients to describe a recent episode of panic or their first ever panic attack. Box 5.9 identifies the information required. It is particularly important to focus on the thoughts or mental images experienced during the episode and any links with specific symptoms.

After discussion of these themes, it often transpires that in an attack the patient is attributing catastrophic interpretations to certain specific sensations, e.g. palpitations linked with a heart attack, dizziness linked to collapse, dry throat and difficulty breathing linked with choking, etc. Examples of specific links between sensations and thoughts are given in Box 5.10.

The therapist elicits the thoughts associated with the onset and maintenance of the reaction by asking: 'At that point, what went through your mind?', 'What was the worst thing you thought might happen?'.

Modifying cognitions. Once important links have been identified between particular bodily sensations and thoughts, the individual is encouraged

Panic diary

Date and time	Situation	Rate severity (0–100)	Bodily sensations	Negative interpretation (rate belief 0–100)	Rational response (rerate belief 0–100)

Figure 5.5 Panic diary.

Date and time	Situation	Rate severity (0–100)	Bodily sensations	Negative interpretation (rate belief 0–100)	Rational response (rerate belief 0–100)
11.9.98 11 a.m.	At home, alone	70	Palpitations, breathless, tight chest	I am having a heart attack I will die alone (80)	It's just anxiety + overbreathing. I've had this before and not died. I know it goes away when I distract myself which shows it's not a heart attack. Maybe I ran up those stairs too fast. (20)
12.9.98	No attacks today				
13.9.98 8.15 a.m.	In the bathroom	60	Feeling faint, unreal sensation, breathless	I'm going to collapse (70)	No I'm not! My pulse is racing and my blood pressure is up. You need a blood pressure drop to faint. I simply feel faint because adrenaline is making more blood go to my muscles. Even though I feel danger, there is none. (5)
2.00 p.m.	Shopping	40	Dizzy, breathless	" " " " (40)	

Figure 5.6 Example of a completed panic diary.

Box 5.9 Information gained from the panic patient

• the circumstances in which the panic occurred
• the bodily sensations experienced
• the behaviour associated with the panic (escape, avoidance, distraction)
• the person's thoughts immediately before and during the panic episode
• any circumstances where an attack is more/less likely

Box 5.10 Examples of specific links between sensations and thoughts

Sensation	Thought/interpretation
Palpitations/heart racing	This is a heart attack; there is something seriously wrong with my heart
Breathlessness	I am going to stop breathing, suffocate and die
Faintness/dizziness	I will faint/fall over/pass out
Unusual thoughts, difficulty thinking	I am going mad

---

to generate more appropriate responses to these sensations, attributing them correctly to their own heightened awareness and the physiological effects of anxiety.

The techniques used to modify these thoughts are common to cognitive therapy for other emotional disorders: search for alternative explanations; considering how other people would interpret the situation; inclusion of otherwise ignored facts; rejecting misleading 'facts' which are being believed; and trying to estimate the probability that the feared catastrophic event will actually take place. The therapist trains the individual to ask questions of themselves during the panic episodes, the most common of which include:

• What evidence do I have for/against this thought?

• Is there an alternative explanation for the situation?

- How can my new understanding of the effects of anxiety on my body help me explain what's happening?

The use of a panic diary will enable them to continue this work outside therapy sessions. An example of a completed diary is shown in Figure 5.6. A panic diary sheet is also included for your use in Appendix 2.

Belief ratings as used in the panic diary are an effective method of monitoring the patient's success in challenging their irrational beliefs and erroneous interpretations. The patient is asked to rate how much they believe a particular identified thought on a scale from 0 – 'I don't believe it at all' to 100 – 'I am absolutely convinced'. Repeated belief ratings can then be used to monitor progress within and between sessions. It is important that the therapist check that treatment has reduced beliefs in real-life feared situations and not just in the clinic.

Behavioural elements to treatment

Behavioural experiments. As well as discussing evidence for and against patients' negative thoughts, therapists should also devise behavioural assignments that help patients check out the validity of these negative thoughts. The rationale underlying behavioural experiments is that the patient's symptoms are reproduced and then reduced in the clinical situation. This can be one of the most powerful methods of changing beliefs as the patient is actually experiencing the feared situation in a new light.

One particularly common alternative explanation is the notion that the symptoms experienced in a panic attack are the result of **hyperventilation**, rather than the catastrophic causes usually considered by patients. A behavioural experiment to test this hypothesis would consider whether voluntary hyperventilation reproduces the bodily symptoms of panic, and whether training in controlled breathing helps reduce these same symptoms. Around 2 minutes of supervised hyperventilation usually produces symptoms which the patient agrees are similar to their panic sensations. Discussions then revolve around the patient's possible interpretation of these sensations if experienced unexpectedly outside the clinic, and they often appreciate the erroneous catastrophic interpretation they would have generated. Once the patient agrees that it is likely that hyperventilation plays a role in their panic attacks, they can proceed to training in controlled breathing, outlined in the next section. Once they accept that they can start and stop their symptoms by controlling their breathing rate, they are only one step away from reattributing their sensations to hyperventilation rather than some impending medical disaster.

Internal focus of attention sometimes accounts for the bodily sensations which panic patients are prone to misinterpret, and can be used in behavioural experiments. Patients often readily agree that their panicky feelings abate when they are distracted. The question here is: can a person distract themselves from having a heart attack, or other medical catastrophes, such as a brain tumour or loss of consciousness?

Breathing retraining. Controlling the rate of breathing is one of the most important techniques the patient can learn to prevent panic getting out of control. The '6-second breath' is explained in detail in Chapter 9 along with other useful anxiety-management techniques. As stated previously, patients who hyperventilate may be helped by rebreathing expired air from a large paper bag in order to increase their concentration of carbon dioxide in the alveoli.

Relaxation training. One of the simplest ways of achieving relaxation is through planning enjoyable and relaxing activities, and planning breaks in busy schedules. Many patients also benefit from more formal training in relaxation techniques. Progressive muscular relaxation training is detailed in Chapter 9. The rationale of using relaxation to control panic symptoms is similar to its use in general anxiety; relaxation reduces physiological arousal, thus reducing the frequency and intensity of symptoms liable to catastrophic misinterpretation. As with breathing techniques, relaxation should be presented as a skill to be learnt through repeated practice with the aim of being able to use it in situations at the onset of panic. In addition, relaxation is valuable as it enables patients to feel they have some control over their symptoms.

Exposure. Within panic disorder, three types of avoidance can be distinguished: firstly, avoidance of specific situations (e.g. social events, travelling on public transport, crowds, shopping); secondly, avoidance of activities that may bring on feared sensations (e.g. exercise); thirdly, avoidance strategies used once symptoms begin (so-called 'safety behaviours', e.g. holding onto solid objects when feeling faint).

All three forms of avoidance maintain patient's negative beliefs and therefore it is important that the therapist encourages patients to enter situations avoided previously in order to 'test out' their fears. Firstly, avoidance behaviours are identified and then subjected to planned and systematic exposure exercises. The methods involved, i.e. graded hierarchies and behavioural tests, are illustrated in Chapters 3 and 4 (*see* Figures 3.3–3.5). Patients are encouraged to expose themselves to feared situations repeatedly and in a graded fashion, whilst relaxed. During these 'behavioural tests or experiments', the patient's habitual maladaptive cognitions are challenged and hopefully modified. Their predictions of impending catastrophe are almost always wrong, giving the opportunity for the patient to generate balanced, alternative interpretations. Monitoring sheets for this are included in Appendix 2.

Preventing relapse. Towards the end of therapy, the sessions focus on education, self-reliance and anticipating future setbacks. The time between sessions is increased gradually and the patient is expected to take over the therapist's role in planning their own exposure experiments, proving their grasp of the techniques involved and identifying which skills have been most effective for them. The therapist ensures that they are able to continue independently as well as having an understanding of the type of future situations which may precipitate setbacks (e.g. stresses or conflicts, losses or bereavements, episodes of ill health), and ways of dealing with these.

It is important for the patient to know that they can regain contact for continued help should the problem become unmanageable. 'Booster sessions' are generally successful in maintaining treatment effects over time. Some patients find it useful to write out a plan of action if the panic should recur. An example is provided in Box 5.11.

Box 5.11 Patient's plan of action for setbacks

What to do if my panic returns

- If I notice that I am becoming increasingly sensitive to my heartbeat and starting to have frightening thoughts and images:
  - restart my daily recordings, trying to find out what may be triggering the thoughts
  - once I know the triggers, set down the evidence for and against at least two alternative explanations and make plans to test these out
- If I find myself starting to avoid situations for reasons of fear, that is the surest sign that I need to:
  - enter those situations repeatedly and
  - remain there for increasing periods until the panic symptoms disappear

---

Appendix 5A

ICD-10 diagnostic criteria for panic disorder

A The individual experiences recurrent panic attacks that are not consistently associated with a specific situation or object, and which often occur spontaneously (i.e. the episodes are unpredictable). The panic attacks are not associated with marked exertion or with exposure to dangerous or life-threatening situations.

B A panic attack is characterised by all of the following:

- it is a discrete episode of intense fear or discomfort

- it starts abruptly

- it reaches a maximum within a few minutes and lasts at least some minutes

- at least four of the symptoms listed below must be present, one of which must be from items a–d.

   - Autonomic arousal symptoms:
      (a) palpitations, pounding heart, or accelerated heart rate
      (b) sweating
      (c) trembling or shaking
      (d) dry mouth (not due to other cause).

   - Symptoms involving chest and abdomen:
      (e) difficulty breathing
      (f) feeling of choking
      (g) chest pain or discomfort
      (h) nausea or abdominal distress (e.g. churning in stomach).

   - Symptoms involving mental state:
      (i) feeling dizzy, unsteady, faint or light-headed
      (j) derealisation or depersonalisation
      (k) fear of losing control, 'going crazy' or passing out
      (l) fear of dying.

   - General symptoms:
      (m) hot flushes or cold chills
      (n) numbness or tingling sensations.

C Most common exclusion criteria are organic mental disorder, physical cause or schizophrenia, mood or somatoform disorders.

DSM-IV criteria for panic attacks

A discrete period of intense fear or discomfort, in which four or more of the following symptoms develop abruptly and peak within 10 minutes:

- palpitations, pounding heart or accelerated heart rate
- sweating
- trembling or shaking
- sensations of shortness of breath or smothering
- feeling of choking
- chest pain or discomfort
- nausea or abdominal distress
- feeling dizzy, unsteady, light-headed or faint
- derealisation or depersonalisation
- fear of losing control or going crazy
- fear of dying
- numbness or tingling sensations
- chills or hot flushes.

DSM-IV criteria for panic disorder (without agoraphobia)

A   Both 1 and 2:

1   recurrent unexpected panic attacks (see above)

2   at least one of the attacks has been followed by 1 month or more of at least one of the following:

- persistent concern about having additional attacks

- worry about the implications of the attack or its consequences (e.g. losing control, having a heart attack or going crazy)
- significant change in behaviour related to the attacks.

B Absence of agoraphobia.

C Panic attacks are not due to the direct physiological effects of a substance (e.g. a drug of abuse or medication) or a general medical condition (e.g. hyperthyroidism).

D Panic attacks are not better accounted for by another mental disorder such as social phobia, specific phobia, obsessive-compulsive disorder, post-traumatic stress disorder or separation anxiety disorder.

Panic disorder – F41.0

Adapted from WHO (1996)

Presenting complaints

Patients may present with one or more physical symptoms (e.g. chest pain, dizziness, shortness of breath). Further enquiry shows the full pattern described below.

Diagnostic features

- Unexplained attacks of anxiety or fear that begin suddenly, develop rapidly and may last only a few minutes.
- The attacks often occur with physical symptoms such as palpitations, chest pain, sensations of choking, churning stomach, dizziness, feelings of unreality or fear of personal disaster (losing control or going mad, heart attack, sudden death).
- An attack often leads to fear of another attack and avoidance of places where attacks have occurred. Patients may avoid exercise or other activities that may produce physical sensations similar to those of a panic attack.

Differential diagnosis

- Many medical conditions may cause symptoms similar to panic attacks (arrhythmia, cerebral ischaemia, coronary disease, thyrotoxicosis). History and physical examination should be sufficient to exclude many of these.

- If attacks occur only in specific feared situations, see *Phobic disorders – F40.*

- If low or sad mood is also present, see *Depression – F32#.*

Panic disorder – F41.0: management guidelines

Essential information for patient and family

- Panic is common and can be treated.

- Anxiety often produces frightening physical sensations. Chest pain, dizziness or shortness of breath are not necessarily signs of a physical illness: they will pass when anxiety is controlled.

- Panic anxiety also causes frightening thoughts (fear of dying, a feeling that one is going mad or will lose control). These also pass when anxiety is controlled.

- Mental and physical anxiety reinforce each other. Concentrating on physical symptoms will increase fear.

- A person who withdraws from or avoids situations where attacks have occurred will only strengthen his/her anxiety.

Counselling of patient and family

- Advise the patient to take the following steps if a panic attack occurs:
  - stay where you are until the attack passes
  - concentrate on controlling anxiety, not on physical symptoms
  - practice slow, relaxed breathing. Breathing too deeply or rapidly (hyperventilation) can cause some of the physical symptoms of panic. Controlled breathing will reduce physical symptoms
  - tell yourself that this is a panic attack and that frightening thoughts and sensations will soon pass. Note the time passing on your watch. It may feel like a long time but it will be only a few minutes.

- Identify exaggerated fears which occur during panic (e.g. patient reminds him/herself, 'I am not having a heart attack. This is a panic attack, and it will pass in a few minutes')..

- Discuss ways to challenge these fears during panic (e.g. patient reminds him/herself, 'I am not having a heart attack. This is a panic attack, and it will pass in a few minutes').

- Self-help groups may help the patient manage panic symptoms and overcome fears.

Medication

- Many patients will benefit from counselling and will not need medication.

- If attacks are frequent and severe, or if the patient is significantly depressed, antidepressants may be helpful (e.g., imipramine 25 mg at night increasing to 100–150 mg at night after 2 weeks).

- For patients with infrequent and limited attacks, short-term use of anti-anxiety medication may be helpful (lorazepam 0.5–1.0 mg up to three times a day). Regular use may lead to dependence and is likely to result in the return of panic symptoms when discontinued.

- Avoid unnecessary tests or medications.

Specialist consultation

- Consider consultation if severe attacks continue after the above treatments.

- Referral for cognitive and behavioural psychotherapies, if available, may be effective for patients who do not improve.

- Panic commonly causes physical symptoms. Avoid unnecessary medical consultation.

6
Acute stress and adjustment disorders

Everybody is affected by stress to some degree at various times; patients complain of it, doctors diagnose it and medical work seems to generate it. But scepticism persists about its meaning, its measurement and its management. So what is it? From a general perspective, stress is a fashionable term denoting usually disagreeable stimuli. It also encompasses the physiological, behavioural and subjective responses to these stimuli.

Defining stress

Despite much scientific and medical research concerned with stress and its effects, none of this intriguing work adequately explains variability in individual responses, disease specificity or the onset of disease. Stress has been implicated in a variety of illnesses including chronic fatigue, peptic ulcers, irritable bowel syndrome, hypertension, angina pectoris and myocardial infarction, strokes, migraine, drug and alcohol addiction, asthma and diabetes (McGlone, 1998). Nevertheless, stress is still very poorly defined in medical circles.

It is therefore worth reflecting on the origins of the word 'stress' in order to appreciate how the term may best be used. It derives from the Latin *stringere*, meaning to 'draw tight', which clearly has a precise meaning as applied to certain materials. The 'elastic' in humans is loosely represented by the neuroendocrine system, when this is 'drawn tight' the tension produces characteristic changes, such as an increase in adrenaline and cortisol, which reflect the biological response to stress. However, whilst ropes and string may be capable of sustained tension, humans usually are not.

Mechanisms of stress

For the purposes of this chapter, stressful factors acting on an individual will be termed *stressors*, and the response of the individual will be termed *stress*. As mentioned, the biological response to stressors involves the neuroendocrine system, which in turn affects the body's physical organs, immune status and emotional control. Importantly, psychological interpretation of the environment affects this biological response, and biological complications of stress may also lead to psychological distress. Hence, primates kept in captivity show markedly increased systemic corticosteroid levels, in addition to disturbed and dysfunctional behaviour. This relationship between biological and psychological factors, viewed as a vicious circle, is shown graphically in Figure 6.1.

The greater the personal meaning attached to stress, such as the loss of a close friend or relative, and the greater the number of stressors, the more likely the occurrence of complications. However, a certain amount of stress may be desirable, if it provides the stimulation and motivation to overcome obstacles in pursuit of a goal; in this respect, there are some people who seem to thrive on stress, and the ability to perceive or withstand stress varies widely. Generally, people try to keep their thoughts, emotions and relationships in a steady, comfortable state. When these are disrupted by outside forces (stressors) the person must act or cope in some way to try and restore the 'comfortable state', thereby maintaining homeostasis. This behavioural adjustment represents a coping strategy, which if successful restores the steady state; if not, continued stress results.

Life events

Since the 1960s psychiatrists and social scientists have recognised the importance of major life changes in producing a variety of illnesses and, in particular, mental health problems. Such life changes are called 'life events' and include divorce, separation, bereavement, redundancy and moving house (*see* Box 6.1). Life events may produce various stress responses, and in some cases they may precipitate an episode of illness such as major depression. The nature of the response is partly determined by the significance the life event holds for the individual. Thus, moving home or even country may be positive for one person, but undesirable for another, particularly if they perceive that the move is forced upon them.

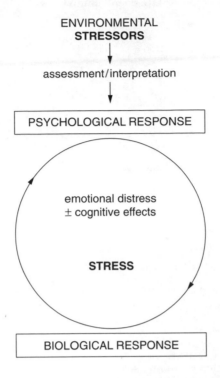

ENVIRONMENTAL
STRESSORS

assessment/interpretation

PSYCHOLOGICAL RESPONSE

emotional distress
± cognitive effects

STRESS

BIOLOGICAL RESPONSE

sympathetic overactivity
hypercortisilaemia
immune impairment

Figure 6.1 Mechanisms of 'stress'.

Life events tend to be particularly stressful when they are:

- in conflict with other important demands
- unpredictable or uncontrollable
- cumulative
- unavoidable
- unfamiliar
- intense or prolonged
- inevitable.

Box 6.1   Holmes and Rahe's hassles scale

Life events and stress

Life event	Stress rating
Death of a spouse	100
Divorce or marital separation	73
Jail term	63
Death of close family member	63
Personal injury or illness	53
Marriage	50
Loss of job	47
Moving house	45
Marital reconciliation	45
Retirement	45
Serious illness of family member	44
Pregnancy	40
Sexual difficulties	39
Birth of a new child	39
Change of job	39
Financial problems	38
Death of a close friend	37
Increase in family disharmony	35
High mortgage	31
Legal action over debt	30
Change in work responsibilities	29
Children leaving home	29
Trouble with in-laws	29
Outstanding personal achievement	28
Spouse begins or stops work	26
Children beginning or ending school	26
Change in living conditions	25
Revision of personal habits	24
Trouble with boss	23
Change in work hours or conditions	20
Change in children's school	20
Change in recreation or leisure pursuits	19
Change in church activities	19
Change in social activities	18
Small mortgage or loan	17
Change in sleeping habits	16
Change in contact with family	15
Change in eating habits	15
Holidays	13
Christmas	12
Minor violations of the law	11

Scoring:

Below 60	– A life unusually free of stress
60–80	– Normal amount of stress
80–100	– Stress in life rather high
100+	– Under serious stress at home, work or both

This exercise is not meant to be taken too seriously – just to give an idea of the various sources of stress in our modern lives.

Recognising stress

Swept along, with too much to do, too little time, and unable to relax, stressed people become exhausted until, failing to cope, they reach breaking-point. Four main types of stress can be recognised:

- acute time limited (e.g. awaiting surgery)
- sequential – one event initiating others that occur over a period (e.g. bereavement)
- chronic intermittent (e.g. conflicts with neighbours)
- chronic (e.g. being disabled).

The more intense the stress, such as loss of a loved one, and the greater the magnitude of stress or number of stresses, the more likely may be the occurrence of diverse ill-effects. At the same time, some people seem to flourish on stress. A certain amount of stress appears desirable to give the stimulation and motivation to overcome obstacles that may prevent us reaching our goals, or to alleviate boredom. The ability to perceive or withstand stress appears to vary widely.

'Warning signs' include:

- irritability
- changes in sleep and eating patterns
- difficulty concentrating and making decisions
- worrying or getting angry about trivia.

Clearly, the symptoms of stress are fairly non-specific (as are, for example, the symptoms of early lung cancer) and attempts have been made to 'tighten up' the definition of stress disorders in recent classifications. One method of restricting the use of the term within medical settings is to confine it to categories from standard diagnostic classifications. The ICD-10 contains a list of reactions to severe stress and adjustment disorders. The main features of these disorders are outlined below (the research diagnostic criteria are given in the Appendix to this chapter).

Acute stress reaction (ICD-10; F43.0)

This is a transient disorder that develops in an individual, without any other apparent mental disorder, in response to exceptional physical and mental stress and which usually subsides within hours or days. Individual vulnerability and coping capacity play a role in the occurrence and severity of acute stress reactions. The symptoms show a typically mixed and changing picture, and include an initial state of 'daze' with some constriction of the field of consciousness and narrowing of attention, inability to comprehend stimuli, and disorientation. This state may be followed either by further withdrawal from the surrounding situation (to the extent of a dissociative stupor) or by agitation and overactivity (flight reaction or fugue). Autonomic signs of anxiety (tachycardia, sweating, flushing) are commonly present. The symptoms usually appear within minutes of the impact of the stressful stimulus or event, and disappear within 2–3 days (often within hours). Partial or complete amnesia for the episode may be present. If the symptoms persist, a change of diagnosis should be considered. (From International Classification of Diseases 10th Edition, WHO, 1994.) The features of an acute stress reaction are given in Box 6.2.

Adjustment disorder (ICD-10; F43.2)

A state of subjective distress and emotional disturbance, usually interfering with social functioning and performance, arising in the

---

Box 6.2 Features of acute stress reaction

- Transient disorder (hours or days)
- Response to exceptional stress
- Autonomic signs of anxiety   – tachycardia
  – sweating
  – flushing
- Mixed picture, *may* include   – initial daze
  – withdrawal
  – overactivity
  – stupor
  – flight/fugue
  – amnesia

period of adaptation to a significant life change or a stressful life event. The stressor may have affected the integrity of the individual's social network (bereavement, separation) or the wider system of social supports and values (migration, refugee status), or represented a major developmental transition or crisis (going to school, becoming a parent, failure to attain a cherished personal goal, retirement). Individual predisposition or vulnerability plays an important role in the risk of occurrence and the shaping of the manifestations of adjustment disorders, but it is nevertheless assumed that the condition would not have arisen without the stressor.

The manifestations vary and include depressed mood, anxiety or worry (or a mixture of these), a feeling of inability to cope, plan ahead or continue in the present situation, as well as some degree of disability in the performance of daily routines. Conduct disorders may be an associated feature, particularly in adolescents. The predominant feature may be a brief or prolonged depressive reaction, or a disturbance of other emotions and conduct. (From International Classification of Diseases, 10th Edition, WHO, 1994.) The features of adjustment disorder are given in Box 6.3.

Box 6.3   Features of adjustment disorder

- A state of subjective distress, during adaptation to life event
- Arises within a month and lasts up to 6 months
- Stressors: – social, e.g. bereavement, separation, experiences, migration
                     – developmental, e.g. starting school, parenthood, retirement
- Symptoms: – depressed mood, anxiety or worry (or a mixture of these)
                     – inability to cope, or plan ahead
                     – disability in the performance of daily routines
                     – conduct disorders in adolescents

Management of stress

As has been illustrated, the two broad categories of stress disorder are acute stress reaction and adjustment disorder; both of these are responses to life events and may be seen as an extreme response to the kind of events faced by most people at some time in their lives. The ideal response to such events is to somehow come to terms with the changes imposed, thereby effectively 'taking control' of life again through a process of *adaptation*. Such adjustment often occurs without coming to the attention of doctors, and is usually the result of personal resolve, coupled with family and social support.

However, where a particularly vulnerable or severely stressed individual is unable to make the required adjustment, they may present to a doctor or other health professional. In these circumstances it is necessary to assess the degree of stress, the patient's ability to cope and the availability of any family and social support.

The very nature of these disorders is that they are time limited, and liable to change considerably over time. Hence, management tends to be 'ad hoc' and tailored to the prevailing circumstances. To illustrate these concepts, an example of acute stress reaction is described in Box 6.4.

From this example of acute stress reaction, it is clear that appropriate assessment led to adequate management. Initially she was found in a 'fugue' state and was amnestic for the preceeding events, so she was kept in a place of safety until transferred for further assessment. Later, although distressed, she was able to account for her situation, and the availability of caring family permitted her safe discharge. No medication was required and she made a 'spontaneous' recovery with no evidence of lasting ill effects.

However, had there been no available support, the patient may have required some form of professional 'crisis intervention' and possibly some sedation (e.g. 5 mg oral diazepam) if severely agitated. The most valuable intervention is support and safety, which clearly need not mean admission to hospital. If symptoms had persisted for substantially longer than 3 days, then reassessment may suggest an adjustment disorder, which may be characterised by anxiety, depression or a mixture of the two.

The same principles of management can be applied to adjustment disorder, an example of which is provided in the case history in Box 6.5 (please read before continuing with the main text).

This example of adjustment disorder illustrates exposure to a life change which may produce symptoms akin to depression, anxiety or both. If the GP had merely prescribed hypnotics, this may simply have masked the underlying problems, which were eventually 'exposed' during the natural history of the disorder. The depressive symptoms may have merited medication, but the personal disclosure revealed clear social precipitants which marked this as an adjustment disorder. Adapting to the situation by 'coming clean' was extremely hard for

Box 6.4 Case history – acute stress reaction

A 23-year-old female student was found wandering late at night in the secure area of a naval installation. The police detained her in custody and she was initially assessed by the forensic medical examiner (FME). He observed that her hair was cropped, she was wearing very little and was unable to account for her actions. She knew her name, but did not know where she was or how she had ended up there. In her jeans' pocket was some money, a photograph and a student card, which enabled some background information to be sought. She was evidently from a university over 100 miles from where she was found, but given the time of night the FME referred her to the on-call psychiatrist at the local hospital, where she was admitted overnight.

The following day she was able to say where she was from, and further enquiries at the university revealed that she was a medical student who had failed her final exams. She was transferred that day to her own local psychiatric service; when she arrived, she was tearful and distracted, but was able to recall most of the previous day's events.

After discovering that she had failed her exams she had gone to see her boyfriend, who disclosed that he wanted to end their relationship. She vaguely recalled that after this she walked into town and headed for the train station, but was unable to recall further details. The assessing doctor found her to be distressed and overtalkative, still a little disorientated, but apparently gaining in insight and wanting to see her father. Her family were contacted and a few hours later she was discharged home, with the recommendation that she see her own GP if things did not settle down over the next few days. In the event, no follow-up was required and the young woman successfully graduated the following year.

the patient, but had his wife rejected him he may at least have had somewhere to start from, rather than the hopeless predicament he was caught in. The 'cure' in this case simply involved counselling and supporting the patient through a process of adaptation.

Box 6.5   Case history – adjustment disorder

A 49-year-old businessman presented to his GP with disturbed sleep for 6 weeks; he had marked delay in getting to sleep (by several hours) and even when he did sleep 'normally' he never felt refreshed. He felt so tired that he could not enjoy any usually pleasurable activity, and he was emotionally 'worn out' and irritable. The GP gently resisted his demands for sleeping tablets, enquiring about 'other things' that were going on in the man's life, but the patient promptly left the surgery.

A few days later he presented himself to the accident and emergency department, where he saw the duty psychiatrist and was admitted with a possible diagnosis of depression and started on antidepressants. Whilst on the psychiatric ward he disclosed his circumstances to the occupational therapist. Two months previously he had borrowed a substantial sum of money from his wife in order to keep his business afloat. However, business spontaneously picked up, and instead of returning the money he went on an expensive cruise with his mistress, who then left him. On his return, business was worse than ever and he felt unable to tell his wife what had happened. He now faced bankruptcy and loneliness and could not see a way out of his situation.

By now feeling hopeless and suicidal, he was eventually persuaded by the ward staff to tell his wife what had happened, on the basis that seemingly little further harm could be done to his future even if she rejected him. Shortly afterwards, there was a moving 'scene' on the ward when the couple spent some time together and were dramatically reconciled. A few days later the patient was discharged, with outpatient follow-up. Three months later, the man had completely lost his business, but was nevertheless enjoying a new quality of married life, his sleep and emotional disturbances were cured, and antidepressant medication was stopped.

Assessment of stress

The stress disorders addressed in the present chapter are clearly related to life events or environmental change, and the primary goal of assessment is to understand the symptoms in terms of such circumstances. In the case history given in Box 6.5 (adjustment disorder) the GP

Box 6.6 Eliciting 'other things' in stress disorders

Time   – be prepared to offer the patient another appoint-
              ment or bring them back after surgery

Observe   – non-verbal communication

Listening   – be *seen* to listen

Questions   – 'Is there anything else troubling you?'
            – 'Did anything else bring you to the surgery?'
            – 'How are you getting on with your partner?'
            – 'How are you managing with the children?'
            – 'How are you getting on at work?'
            – 'Have you been drinking more than usual?'

These suggestions may be remembered by the acronym **T O L Q**
(TALK)

---

made a gallant effort to elicit 'other things' going on in the patient's life.
Suitable ways of assessing these other areas of concern to the patient are
summarised in Box 6.6.

In the context of a trusting and sympathetic doctor–patient relationship, the approach outlined in Box 6.6 will usually allow the patient to
divulge quite painful or embarrassing personal circumstances. However,
the clinician should be aware of potential sinister complications
associated with stress, such as the abuse of alcohol and drugs. The
complications of stress are summarised in Box 6.7.

Box 6.7 Complications of stress

• alcohol abuse, see Chapter 9 – Self-help
• drugs including cigarettes, see Chapter 9 – Self-help
• risk of anxiety/depression
• risk of physical illness, e.g. chronic fatigue, peptic ulcers,
  irritable bowel syndrome, hypertension, angina pectoris and
  myocardial infarction, strokes, migraine, asthma and diabetes

Treatment of stress

The very nature of stress is that it is predominantly a response to environmental stressors, and ultimately its cure is effected either by adaptation, problem solving or change of environment. Where change of circumstances is not possible, the ideal course of action is some form of support and counselling, either informal (family and friends) or formal (health professionals). It cannot be overemphasised that most stress is self-limiting and hence is not seen by doctors. The treatment of stress in this chapter is therefore confined to those patients who seek medical help.

Medical treatment of stress

Most cases of adjustment disorder and acute stress reaction will respond adequately to measures of appropriate adaptation. However, in cases which are complicated by severe symptoms, or drug and alcohol excess, conventional medical intervention may be required. The guiding principle is therefore to treat according to the predominant symptoms, and suggested pharmaceutical agents are summarised in Box 6.8. It should be emphasised, however, that drugs should only be used in the treatment of stress which is severe and debilitating, and should not be seen as a 'panacea' for stress.

Psychological aspects of treatment – a psychological model of stress

As proposed previously, stress is best described as part of a complex and dynamic system of transaction between the individual and their environment. According to the psychological model illustrated in Figure 6.2, stress arises when there is an *imbalance* between the perceived demand of a situation and the individual's perception of their ability to meet that demand. The crucial aspect here is not their *actual* capability, but whether they *perceive* themselves able to cope with the demand. Hence, *cognitive appraisal* of the factors involved can become the focus for psychological treatment, enabling individuals under extreme stress to more accurately appraise both the potentially stressful situation and their ability to cope with it.

Box 6.8 Drugs for severe stress disorders

Acute stress reaction
- Marked agitation – lorazepam; 1 mg orally prn up to 4 mg max. daily for 1 or 2 days only* **or**
  – diazepam; 2–5 mg orally prn up to 15 mg daily for a few days only* **or**
  – thioridazine; 25–100 mg orally prn up to 400 mg daily

Adjustment disorder
- Marked agitation – as above
- Depressive or anxiety symptoms – SSRI (according to British National Formulary recommendations) to be reviewed monthly
- Insomnia – zolpidem†; 5–10 mg orally at night **or**
  – zopiclone†; 3.75–7.5 mg orally at night

*High potential for dependence.
†Modest potential for dependence.

Implications for treatment

Clearly, the demands placed upon individuals may in truth be beyond their ability to cope with. Accurate reappraisal will then ideally motivate the person to either undertake action to reduce the actual demands (e.g. negotiation with work managers, communication with spouse) and/or to increase their coping skills (e.g. seek social support, implement time- and stress-management techniques, relaxation and leisure activities). Guidelines on problem solving, relaxation and other anxiety-management techniques are provided elsewhere in this text and patient material is included in Chapter 9.

Counselling sessions may be indicated where it seems that the individual does possess the necessary abilty and coping skills to manage their situation, but a lack of self-confidence is holding them back.

CBT is clearly relevant in addressing stress, with the focus on modifying cognitive defences, cognitive reappraisal and developing adaptive behavioural responses. Patients with stress reactions are often

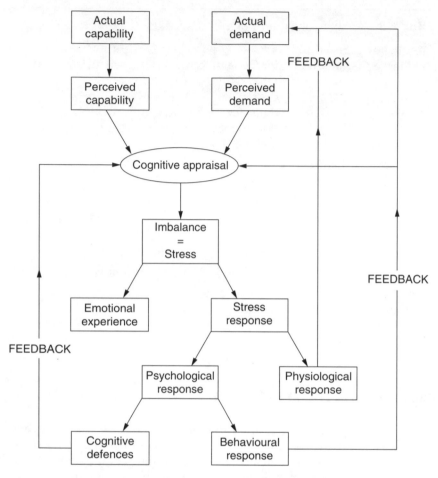

Figure 6.2 Transactional model of stress (from Cox, 1988).

advised to maintain an organised pattern of behaviour based on logical reasoning. Although such a routine and 'mechanical' lifestyle may not have the spontaneity of a more stimulating and flexible way of life, it is undoubtedly more effective in sustaining the person through periods of extreme stress. The reduced need for conscious investment enables the individual to devote their psychological resources and cognitive capacity to the higher purpose of managing their current problems.

Other behavioural strategies include scheduling of pleasurable activities and exercise. As the physiological response to stress can cause 'wear and tear' on the body and physical complications, active behavioural coping is an effective method of limiting this process. Paced exercise has been found to reduce catecholamine levels in stressed individuals and such a simple intervention is readily accepted by patients as a means of 'releasing tension'.

If the stress persists despite such interventions, the individual may be advised to consider more radical environmental changes (e.g. taking a career break, committment to relationships), sometimes requiring drastic prioritising of 'life goals'. Hence, it may be necessary to decide between marital harmony and career objectives. Clearly, such important life decisions should not be taken without due consideration; some actions taken when under stress are later regretted.

Self-help materials and information are provided in Chapter 9 for patients' own use.

Appendix 6A

ICD-10 criteria for adjustment disorders

Diagnostic criteria for adjustment disorders

A   Onset of symptoms must occur within one month of exposure to an identifiable psychosocial stressor, not of an unusual or catastrophic type.

B   The individual manifests symptoms or behaviour disturbance of the types found in any of the affective disorders (F30–F39) (except for delusions and hallucinations), any disorders in F40–F48 (neurotic, stress-related and somatoform disorders) and conduct disorders. Symptoms may be variable in both form and severity.

The predominant feature of the symptoms may be further specified by the use of a fifth character:

F43.20   *Brief depressive reaction.* A transient mild depressive state of a duration not exceeding one month.

F43.21   *Prolonged depressive reaction.* A mild depressive state occurring in response to a prolonged exposure to a stressful situation but of a duration not exceeding two years.

F43.22   *Mixed anxiety and depressive reaction.* Both anxiety and depressive symptoms are prominent, but at levels no greater than those specified for mixed anxiety and depressive disorder (F41.2) or other mixed anxiety disorders (F41.3).

F43.23   *With predominant disturbance of other emotions.* The symptoms are usually of several types of emotion, such as anxiety, depression, worry, tension and anger. Symptoms of anxiety and depression may meet the criteria for mixed anxiety and depressive disorder (F41.2) or for other mixed anxiety disorders (F41.3), but they are not so predominant that other more specific depressive or anxiety disorders can be diagnosed. This category should also be used for reactions in children in whom regressive behaviour, such as bed-wetting or thumb-sucking are also present.

F43.24   *With predominant disturbance of conduct.* The main disturbance is one involving conduct, e.g. an adolescent grief reaction resulting in aggressive or dissocial behaviour.

F43.25 *With mixed disturbance of emotions and conduct.* Both emotional symptoms and disturbances of conduct are prominent features.

F43.28 *With other specified predominant symptoms.* Except in prolonged depressive reaction (F43.21) the symptoms do not persist for more than six months after the cessation of the stress or its consequences. (However, this should not prevent a provisional diagnosis being made if this criterion is not yet fulfilled).

ICD-10 criteria for acute stress reaction

Diagnostic criteria for acute stress reaction

A The patient must have been exposed to an exceptional mental or physical stressor.

B Exposure to the stressor is followed by an immediate onset of symptoms (within one hour).

C Two groups of symptoms are given and the acute stress reaction is graded as:

F43.00 mild; only criterion 1 below is fulfilled

F43.01 moderate; criterion 1 is met and there are any two symptoms from criterion 2

F43.02 severe: either criterion 1 is met and there are any four symptoms from criterion 2, or there is dissociative stupor (*see* F44.2).
1 criteria B, C and D for generalised anxiety disorder (F41.1) are met
2 a withdrawal from expected social interaction
b narrowing of attention
c apparent disorientation
d anger or verbal aggression
e despair or hopelessness
f inappropriate or purposeless overactivity
g uncontrollable and excessive grief judged by local cultural standards.

D If the stressor is transient or can be relieved, the symptoms must begin to diminish after not more than eight hours. If exposure to the stressor continues, the symptoms must begin to diminish after not more than 48 hours.

E   *Most commonly used exclusion clause.* The reaction must occur in the absence of any other concurrent mental or behavioural disorder in ICD-10 (except 41.1, generalised anxiety disorder, and F60, personality disorders), and not within three months of the end of an episode of any other mental or behavioural disorder.

DSM-IV criteria for adjustment disorders

Diagnostic criteria for adjustment disorders

A   The development of emotional or behavioural symptoms in response to an identifiable stressor(s) occurring within three months of the onset of the stressor(s).

B   These symptoms or behaviours are clinically significant as evidenced by either of the following:

1 marked distress that is in excess of what would be expected from exposure to the stressor
2 significant impairment in social or occupational (academic) functioning.

C   The stress-related disturbance does not meet the criteria for another specific Axis I disorder and is not merely an exacerbation of a pre-existing Axis I or Axis II disorder.

D   The symptoms do not represent bereavement.

E   Once the stressor (or its consequences) has been terminated, the symptoms do not persist for more than an additional six months.

Specify if:
Acute: if the disturbance lasts less than six months
Chronic: if the disturbance lasts for six months or longer

Adjustment disorders are coded based on the subtype which is selected according to the predominant symptoms. The specific stressor(s) can be specified on Axis IV.

309.0   With depressed mood
309.24 With anxiety
309.28 With mixed anxiety and depressed mood
309.3   With disturbance of conduct
309.4   With mixed disturbance of emotions and conduct
309.9   Unspecified

DSM-IV criteria for acute stress disorder

Diagnostic criteria for acute stress disorder

A   The person has been exposed to a traumatic event in which both of the following were present:

1 the person experienced, witnessed, or was confronted with an event or events that involved actual or threatened death or serious injury, or a threat to the physical integrity of self or others

2 the person's response involved intense fear, helplessness or horror.

B   Either while experiencing or after experiencing the distressing event, the individual has three (or more) of the following dissociative symptoms:

1 a subjective sense of numbing, detachment or absence of emotional responsiveness

2 a reduction in awareness of his or her surroundings, e.g. 'being in a daze'

3 derealisation

4 depersonalisation

5 dissociative amnesia, i.e. inability to recall an important aspect of the trauma.

C   The traumatic event is persistently re-experienced in at least one of the following ways: recurrent images, thoughts, dreams, illusions, flashback episodes, or a sense of reliving the experience, or distress on exposure to reminders of the traumatic event.

D   Marked avoidance of stimuli that arouse recollections of the trauma, e.g. thoughts, feelings, conversations, activities, places, people.

E   Marked symptoms of anxiety or increased arousal, e.g. difficulty sleeping, irritability, poor concentration, hypervigilance, exaggerated startle response, motor restlessness.

F   The disturbance causes clinically significant distress or impairment in social occupational, or other important areas of functioning or impairs the individual's ability to pursue some necessary task, such as obtaining necessary assistance or mobilising personal resources by telling family members about the traumatic experience.

G   The disturbance lasts for a minimum of two days and a maximum of four weeks and occurs within four weeks of the traumatic event.

H   The disturbance is not due to the direct physiological effects of a substance (e.g. a drug of abuse, a medication) or a general medical condition is not better accounted for by brief psychotic disorder, and is not merely an exacerbation of a pre-existing Axis I or Axis II disorder.

7
Post-traumatic stress disorder

Introduction

Post-traumatic stress disorder (PTSD) has gained international recognition as a psychiatric disorder only recently, appearing in the World Health Organisation's International Classification of Diseases for the first time in 1992 (ICD-10). However, the condition is not new and has existed under various names for centuries, early descriptions following the Great Fire of London in 1666. This century has seen the epithets 'shell shock', 'battle fatigue' and 'combat neurosis' applied to the condition, reflecting its prominence in war, but it is now almost universally known as 'PTSD'.

Definition

The principal features were first described by Kardiner (1941), who saw it as a 'physio-neurosis' involving both physiological and psychological components, and the characteristic features are summarised in Box 7.1. PTSD is essentially a delayed or protracted response to a stressful event (trauma) to a degree sufficiently threatening or catastrophic as to cause marked distress in almost anyone. The protracted response of PTSD involves repeated *reliving* of the trauma through intrusive memories ('flashbacks' and/or nightmares); a sense of emotional *'numbness'* and detachment from other people; *avoidance* of situations reminiscent of the trauma; and also a state of autonomic *hyperarousal* marked by hypervigilance, enhanced startle reaction and insomnia.

> **Box 7.1** Core features of PTSD
>
> - **Exposure** to traumatic event
> - **Avoidance** of reminiscent situations
> - **Reliving** by flashbacks and/or nightmares
> - **Numbness** or sense of detachment from people and surroundings
> - **Hyperarousal** enhanced startle reaction and insomnia
>
> **Aide de memoire** – trauma may **E A R N** Hyperarousal

Aetiology

The trigger for PTSD is exposure to a catastrophic or overwhelmingly threatening event, which may be brief or sustained. However, such exposure alone is insufficient to explain the disorder, as it only occurs in a proportion of those exposed to such trauma. Kulka *et al.* (1990) reviewed the data on Vietnam veterans and found that fewer than 40% of those with high war-zone exposure developed PTSD. Hence, it appears that triggers acting on predisposed individuals contribute to the disorder. In civilian studies triggers are: rape (57%), physical assault (37%) and robbery (28%) (Kilpatrick and Resnick, 1993).

Attempts to characterise such predisposed individuals include: studies of heritability in humans, neurobiological animal models and psychosocial vulnerability factors.

Twin studies have shown that PTSD has a heritability of 0.3, indicating that genetic factors alone make a 30% contribution to the disorder (True *et al.*, 1993). Family studies have shown high rates of alcoholism among siblings, as well as a disturbed childhood marked by poor parent–child relationships, in those developing PTSD. Hence, it becomes clear that the disorder results from traumatic triggers acting on those who are predisposed by virtue of biopsychosocial factors.

Once the trigger has exerted its effects on the vulnerable subject, there appears to follow a neurobehavioural pattern associated with abnormalities of brain function. The available evidence suggests important roles for the following structures: the locus coeruleus, with its noradrenergic fibres projecting widely through the brain; the central nucleus of the amygdala, projecting into the brainstem; and the limbic nuclei, which are involved in emotional arousal.

The natural history of PTSD is characterised by a delay, or latency period, between the trauma and the onset of illness, which may range from days to months. There is some evidence that modulating factors exert an influence during this latency period, which may increase or decrease the likelihood of developing the actual disorder. Factors that increase the risk of illness may occur at a psychobiological level (e.g. an inability to process the somatic memory of the traumatic event) and at a psychosocial level (e.g. negative social attitudes to involvement in an event like rape). Modulating factors that reduce the risk of illness include: positive public opinion (e.g. the welcoming home of 'war heroes' from a popular campaign) and cognitive processing of traumatic events (as may be effected by constructive debriefing).

Aetiology is therefore multifactorial and sequential, and the principal components are summarised diagrammatically in Figure 7.1.

The neurochemistry of memory formation has gained recent prominence in the aetiology of PTSD. It is particularly interesting that

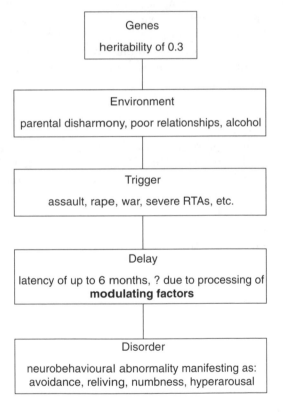

Figure 7.1 The aetiology of PTSD.

unconsciousness following major trauma appears to protect from PTSD, although clinical evidence suggests that there is a sub-group of people who, as a result of not being able to remember the actual traumatic events, develop a particularly refractory form of PTSD characterised by **imagined** memories.

Neurochemistry

Excitation

The principal *excitatory* neurotransmitter in the brain is **glutamate**, which has a central role in memory and consciousness. Glutamatergic neurones ascending from the brainstem to the cortex are disrupted in concussion, presumably as a result of pressure and shearing forces. It is thought that stressors are laid down as memories when they cause enough glutamate release to activate N-methyl-D-aspartate (NMDA) receptors. **Noradrenaline** also contributes to the process of memory formation in the brain, by potentiating the actions of glutamate in the hippocampus. If this exctitatory mechanism is interrupted, as in loss of consciousness, then stressful memories are less likely to be laid down.

Inhibition

Unconsciousness may be produced either by interrupting the excitatory glutamatergic pathways ascending from the brainstem, as outlined above, or by actively increasing inhibition in the brain. GABA is the primary inhibitory neurotransmitter in the brain, and it acts principally on the GABA-A receptor. GABA-ergic drugs, such as benzodiazepines and anaesthetics, act via GABA receptors to render people amnesic or unconscious, depending on the dose. The possibility of using amnestic agents to reduce the risk of PTSD in survivors of severe trauma has been the subject of recent interest.

Epidemiology

Despite the use of increasingly refined diagnostic instruments, there remains a fairly wide estimation of the extent of PTSD in the general population, with a lifetime prevalence of 1–9%; there is little data on gender ratios, but it is clear that illness is by definition, increased following severe trauma and hence there is a proponderence of PTSD in war veterans, who are usually male. There are also high levels of comorbidity, in particular depression, alcohol and substance abuse.

Indeed, the natural history of the 'pure' form of disorder is difficult to elucidate because so many of the sufferers go on to use substances, or develop secondary depression or generalised anxiety. There is ample evidence, however, that the core features of avoidance, hypervigilance, numbing and flashbacks persist for years or decades following the initial trauma. Moreover, Titchener (1985) identifies the resulting detachment from friends and family as the most malignant sequel to PTSD, often accounting for the severe social and psychiatric decline seen in the disorder.

The rates of PTSD following a variety of traumatic 'trigger' events are shown in Box 7.2.

Box 7.2   Rates of PTSD with exposure to different traumas

Vietnam   –   31% men; 27% women

Crimes   –   28% in women victims of any crime
            –   57% completed rape
            –   16% attempted rape
            –   37% aggravated assault
            –   18% robbery
            –   28% burglary

POWs   –   50% → severe PTSD symptoms

Hostages   –   66% → severe – very severe PTSD

Clinical features

The four core clinical features are highlighted in bold in the following description.

The central feature of PTSD is **re-experiencing** the original trauma, in the form of intrusive and unwanted memories. Intrusive memories may take the form of vivid 'flashbacks' during which the subject may feel he or she is reliving the original trauma. Such memories may be triggered by relatively minor stimuli, and Stein (1998) gives the example of Vietnam veterans experiencing intense flashbacks on a rainy day (the monsoon lasts for months in Vietnam). In severe cases the subject actually acts as if he or she were in the midst of the original trauma, the senses assailed by smells, sight and sound associated with the past event. Moreover, intrusive memories may also be experienced during sleep, with distressing nightmares akin to the causal events.

The physiological **hyperarousal** manifests itself as hypervigilance and insomnia. The hypervigilant subject is easily frightened by minor sudden stimuli, owing to an exaggerated startle reflex; an innocent pat on the shoulder from an old acquaintance may provoke a dispropor-tionate jump and cry of intense fear. The subject tends always to be excessively alert as if in readiness for some supposed threat of attack, and appears to over-react to usually innocuous stimuli. Moreover, owing to this marked hypervigilance, the PTSD sufferer finds that sleep onset is delayed, whilst sleep itself is light and easily interrupted, and frequently disturbed by nightmares. The dreaming tends to be repetitious, involving somewhat stereotyped narratives of running away or being attacked, etc. and the content is all too well remembered on waking (in contrast to the nightmares of normal subjects).

The distressing emotions associated with the initial trauma are usually so aversive as to cause the subject to avoid any situations reminiscent of causal events, and which may trigger flashbacks or associated emotions. This core feature of **avoidance** has been well described by Horowitz (1986); the trauma may be followed by a denial phase, during which avoidance is maximal, the individual tending to minimise the role of the initial trauma in causing the present psychological distress. This denial may be accompanied by a general lack of emotional responsiveness, or **numbness**, together with a narrowing of thinking and affect, which results in a reduced ability to experience either pleasure or pain. This in turn may lead to increasing detachment from friends and family, and ultimately to isolation. The clinical features of PTSD are illustrated in the case example given in Box 7.3.

In summary, the clinical features of PTSD are:

- re-experiencing

- hypervigilance

- avoidance

- emotional numbness.

'Positive' and 'negative' symptoms

The clinical features of PTSD have been divided into positive symptoms (re-experiencing and hypervigilance) and negative symptoms (avoid-

> **Box 7.3 Case example of PTSD**
>
> John is a 29-year-old quarry worker who was referred to his GP by
> the occupational health department at his work. Ten months
> previously he had been involved in an accident, at the quarry
> face, in which two of his workmates were killed. The accident was
> reported to be the result of exceptionally heavy rain and therefore
> nobody was considered to be at fault. Nevertheless, since that time
> John had been experiencing nightmares of the scene at the quarry:
> darkness, raining, landslides and screaming, flashing lights and
> blood. During the day he felt increasingly numb and remote from
> what was going on around him; people at work now left him alone
> as he was difficult to engage in conversation, and persistent efforts
> met with silence or angry outbursts. He was jumpy and easily
> startled, and refused to go near the quarry face so that his
> supervisors began to suspect that he was either 'weak' or
> malingering. His girlfriend said he was now a 'different person',
> no longer socialising or enjoying leisure activities like football. At
> clinical assessment he appeared hypervigilant and reported night-
> mares and occasional daytime flashbacks, together with a sense of
> emotional numbness and avoidance of reminders. He also
> admitted to smoking cannabis occasionally (something he had
> never done previously) in order 'to get some peace', particularly at
> night.

ance and emotional numbness). The relevance of this distinction in
symptomatology is that early studies assumed an association between
symptom specificity and drug efficacy; hence, it was found that certain
anticonvulsants were effective in reducing intrusive and arousal
symptoms, but not avoidance. More recent work indicates that selective
SSRIs, in particular fluoxetine, are effective in treating both positive and
negative symptoms in PTSD, and so the distinction is of less importance
in drug therapy.

Differential diagnosis

PTSD shares certain features with a number of psychiatric disorders, in
particular those listed in Box 7.4. Their distinguishing characteristics are
outlined to enable the clinician to arrive at a working diagnosis.

Box 7.4   Differential diagnosis of PTSD
- primary insomnia
- generalised anxiety
- agoraphobia
- agitated depression
- adjustment disorder
- dissociative disorders
- focal epilepsy (TLE)
- stimulant abuse
- malingering

Any of the following may occur chronologically following trauma, but typically are not a direct result of it.

- **Primary insomnia** is frequently seen in the general population. It is distressing and can impair work and social life, but by definition it is not associated with other core features of PTSD.

- **Generalised anxiety** is characterised by persistent anxiety over time, and in various settings. Whilst there may be difficulty with sleep onset and over-arousal, there are no flashback phenomena, and avoidance (if present) is not restricted to 'event stimuli'.

- **Agoraphobia** (Greek *agora* – market) is characterised by symptoms of anxiety associated with crowded places such as shops, and the resulting avoidance is specific to such situations. This has similarities to PTSD, but there is no identifiable precipitating trauma, no flashbacks and no 'numbing' of affect at normal times.

- **Agitated depression** does not typically follow trauma; it manifests as low mood in contrast to 'no' mood in the context of psychomotor agitation which may mimic over-arousal. Although severe cases may feature catastrophic or apocalyptic hallucinations (e.g. 'end of the world' scenes or commentaries) there are no flashbacks.

- **Adjustment disorders** occur following a stressor, although usually less severe than in PTSD. Examples may be the break-up of a relationship or unexpected redundancy, producing a stress reaction which resolves during a period of adaptation (weeks or months). An **acute stress reaction** should have resolved within 4 weeks.

- Flashbacks may occasionally occur in **dissociative disorders**, and more rarely in brief (reactive) psychosis. Rarely, fearful aura or déjà vu associated with partial seizures, of temporal lobe origin, may give rise to flashbacks.

- Finally, vivid flashbacks are also seen in **stimulant abuse**, notably lysergic acid diethylamide (LSD), and M-deoxy-met-amphetamine (MDMA, 'ecstacy'). The Vietnam war again gives rise to examples of the former, with reports of helicopters crashing as a result of pilots having flashbacks of 'acid trips'. Of more contemporary relevance, it is not uncommon for people who use 'ecstacy' at the weekend only, vividly to re-experience nightclub scenes during the week.

Assessment of PTSD

Presentation

Patients may present to their GP weeks or months after a traumatic event, complaining of symptoms ranging from disturbed sleep to marital or relationship problems, yet the sufferer may not volunteer involvement in a trauma. This lack of disclosure may be due to various factors. The individual may be unaware that psychological mechanisms of denial are in operation, or there may be a conscious fear of stigma or censure following rape, for example. Clearly, any core symptoms of PTSD should prompt specific questions in relation to the other symptoms, and in particular to relatively recent (less than 6 months) experience of a life-threatening trauma or situation.

Assessing severity

When patients present for professional help after a traumatic experience, they are likely to disclose the event in the hope of gaining appropriate help and support. The GP is well placed to understand the likely impact of certain tragedies in the community and may readily diagnose PTSD, given the core features already described. However, it is also important to gauge the severity of symptoms and the impact of the disorder on individual functioning, as this information will to some extent influence management. Box 7.5 lists categories of questions that may be asked in assessing the overall severity of PTSD; where a practice counsellor is available, they may be well suited to using the inventory, with a view to supporting milder problems themselves, the more severe cases being referred for specialist intervention. (The complete list of questions is given in the Appendix to this chapter.)

There exists a variety of patient rating scales and structured interviews for the assessment of PTSD and these are summarised in Box 7.6.

Treatment of PTSD

Until relatively recently the mainstay of treatment for PTSD has been psychological together with symptomatic treatment for:

- accompanying problems, such as poor sleep, and

- sequelae, such as substance abuse and relationship difficulties.

This approach is still the most commonly used, but in light of the recent neurochemical findings described above, there is a growing awareness of the role of pharmacotherapy for the underlying biological abnormalities. The following sections deal with biological treatment and psychological intervention.

Pharmacotherapy

In approaching drug treatment for PTSD it should be borne in mind that the disorder has a characteristc natural history. A partly genetically predisposed individual is exposed to a trigger event, there may then follow a latent period of up to 6 months, the core symptoms then begin to manifest, and finally, the established condition may lead to self-medication (alcohol or drugs) and ultimately to social isolation. Treatment must therefore attempt to be relevant to the *phase* of the illness. In view of the phasal nature of PTSD, the drug treatment may be conveniently addressed using the traditional concepts of disease prevention.

Box 7.5 Assessing PTSD at interview

- Traumatic event   – When did it happen?
  - What happened to you exactly?
  - Did you think you were going to die?

- Avoidance   – Do you avoid stituations that remind you of the trauma?
  - Do you avoid these at any cost?

- Re-experiencing   – Do you have nightmares of this or similar events?
  - Can you recall details on waking?
  - When you're awake do you have intrusive thoughts or memories of the trauma?
  - Do you have 'flashbacks' in which you feel as if you're reliving the original trauma?

- Numbness   – Do you feel emotionally cut off from the world around you?
  - Do you feel like a spectator?

- Hyperarousal   – Do you get easily irritated?
  - More so than before the trauma?
  - Do you feel anxious or 'on edge' most of the time?
  - Do you get easily startled or feel 'jumpy' more than before?

- Substance abuse   – Have you been using drugs or alcohol to help you cope?
  - What have you been using, and how much?
  - Is this a problem to you?
  - Is it a problem to those close to you?

- Suicidal ideation   – Have you felt life is not worth living?
  - Have you thought of ending your life?
  - Have you made plans to end your life?
  - Have you started to do things according to that plan?
  - Have you actually made an attempt on your life?

Adapted from Scott and Stradling (1995).

> **Box 7.6**
>
> **Patient rating scales:**
> - PENN Inventory (Hammaberg, 1992)
> - Impact of Events Scale (Horowitz *et al.*, 1979)
>
> **Structured interviews:**
> - CAPS-I, Clinician-Administered PTSD Scale (Blake, 1990)
> - PTSD-I, PTSD-Interview (Watson *et al.*, 1991)
> - SI-PTSD, Structured Interview for PTSD (Davidson *et al.*, 1989)

Primary prevention

Preventing the occurrence of traumatic events is clearly beyond the scope of routine clinical practice; preventing exposure to such events may possibly be achieved through public education with respect to avoiding certain risk-laden situations. Clearly there is no role for pharmacological interventions in primary prevention.

Secondary prevention

Secondary prevention aims to reduce the risk of developing PTSD following exposure to trigger events. Psychological approaches such as early 'debriefing' are considered later. In terms of pharmacotherapy, recent work suggests that immediate post-trauma sedation with benzodiazepines and/or opioids may reduce the intensity of memory formation for the stressor. However, such an approach is still at the research stage, and there is some evidence that conventional amnestic agents, whilst inhibiting anterograde amnesia (after the event), may actually enhance retrograde memory formation (up to and including the event, if conscious).

There is now increasing evidence that, once fully established, the syndrome of PTSD may respond beneficially to treatment with SSRIs. Paroxetine appears to have received most attention in this respect, and current opinion is in favour of a therapeutic trial of the drug at higher doses than would normally be used in the treament of depression.

Core symptoms

In established cases of PTSD, where there is deterioration in social or occupational functioning, it is worthwhile prescribing a SSRI, for example paroxetine or fluoxetine 20 mg rising to 40 mg after 2 weeks. It is advisable to continue SSRI therapy for a minimum of 6 months, or for at least 3 months after the remission of symptoms.

Associated symptoms

The short-acting benzodiazepine **alprazolam** has been shown to be effective in improving anxiety and well-being in PTSD, but it has no effect on the core symptoms (Braun *et al.*, 1990). If used at all, it should be prescribed in divided doses to a maximum of 3 mg daily for a limited period only (usually up to 2 weeks) and withdrawn slowly.

Tertiary prevention

The aim of tertiary prevention is to reduce the complications of the disorder. As already described, the most common sequelae of PTSD are alcohol and drug abuse, and social isolation.

Substance abuse

Self-medication with alcohol and drugs warrants the same therapeutic approach as used in any other setting, and involves a combination of psychotherapeutic (motivational therapy) and pharmacological approaches. Alcohol is the most common substance abused in PTSD, and pharmacotherapy includes **disulfiram** and **acamprosate**. Neither should be given in the absence of some form of structured counselling. Disulfiram inhibits the metabolism of alcohol, resulting in the accumulation of acetaldehyde, which causes intense nausea; its use has largely been superceded by acamprosate, which acts via GABA receptors to reduce craving (*see* British National Formulary for important drug information).

Augmentation drug therapy

Refractory PTSD may respond to certain drugs aimed at specific symptoms. Hence, for example, poor impulse control may respond to lithium and hyperarousal to clonidine. These symptom-specific treatments are summarised in Box 7.7, which provides a summary of drug treatment in PTSD.

Box 7.7   Drug treatment of PTSD

Core symptoms:

- SSRI, e.g. paroxetine 20–40 mg daily for 6 months or fluoxetine 20–40 mg daily for 6 months

Ineffective/poorly tolerated:

- Change to different class of antidepressant at therapeutic dose (see British National Formulary), e.g. TCA, RIMA, MAOI or another SSRI
- Consider specialist referral

Augmentation drug therapy:

- Lithium – poor impulse control
- Carbamazepine – persistent positive symptoms, aggression
- Propranolol – physiological hyperarousal (marked 'jumpiness')
- Clonidine – hyperarousal
- Benzodiazepines – severe anxiety/insomnia (use with caution)

Complications:

- Alcohol abuse – acamprosate 666 mg TDS for 1 year if abstinent.

Adapted from McIvor (1998).

Psychological management of PTSD

Theoretical models of PTSD

Many theoretical models have been proposed in attempts to organise observed patterns of reactions in PTSD and to explain their development and maintenance. The major contributions to our understanding and treatment of PTSD are outlined in Box 7.8.

Box 7.8   Theoretical models of PTSD

- **Psychodynamic**: Freud (1939) observed the two major character-istics of repetition (re-experiencing) and denial (avoidance)

- **Information processing**: Horowitz (1976) proposed that adjust-ment to a traumatic event requires incorporation into existing cognitive schemas about the self and the world. To accomplish this integration, traumatic memories are repeated in 'active memory' in an attempt to regulate information processing

- **Biological**: Van der Kolk and colleagues (1984) observed that PTSD is similar to the animal model of 'inescapable shock' and postulated that symptoms result from changes in neurotrans-mitter activity. They paid particular attention to noradrenergic overactivity and depletion systems

- **Behavioural**: Keane and colleagues (1985) developed a simple two-factor learning theory, whereby any stimulus associated with the trauma becomes (via classical conditioning) capable of eliciting the trauma response. Avoidance develops to escape or prevent this response. Behavioural models continue to evolve with new proposals being frequently added to explain factors such as vulnerability and social support

- **Cognitive processing**: Creamer and co-workers (1992) propose five stages required for successful integration of the trauma: objective exposure, network formation, intrusion, avoidance and recovery. Jones and Barlow (1992) expand this model, incorpor-ating a feedback loop in which hyperarousal, hypervigilance and narrowing of attention serve to increase intrusive thoughts and re-experiencing

Psychological components of PTSD

The psychological reactions exhibited in PTSD reflect an extreme response to a severe stressor including:

- increased anxiety or heightened physiological arousal (can include outbursts of extreme anger)

- hypervigilance ('jumpiness', unrealistic fear of danger)

- re-experiencing phenomena (flashbacks, nightmares)
- avoidance of stimuli associated with the trauma (can include agoraphobia)
- a numbing of emotional responses (thought to be a protective mechanism).

A symptomatic approach to treatment

The following cognitive-behavioural strategies have been adapted for use by non-specialist health professionals, to guide their input and care of people with PTSD in the community. However, should the patient fail to improve, or when symptoms are particularly protracted or severe, then it is advisable to refer the patient to a specialist in the field.

Intrusive imagery/thoughts

Intrusive imagery or thoughts comprise the hallmark of PTSD. They pose a threat to the individual's sense of control and predictability, images arising unbidden and without warning. Psychogenic amnesia may occur in extreme and rare cases, where the patient becomes dissociated from normal everyday functioning, may enter into a fugue state, assuming another identity and name, without any recall of the past. More commonly, however, the patient may experience depersonalisation, feeling 'not themselves', their thoughts and mental life seemingly out of their own control.

These symptoms, and the extent to which they dominate a person's life, vary between individuals and generally improve with time. Four strategies are used to help the patient cope with intrusion; containment, desensitisation, cognitive restructuring and 'balancing out'.

Containment. Typically, patients want to be rid of their intrusive imagery or thoughts and attempt to avoid thinking about the trauma. But, paradoxically, the harder they try not to recall what happened, the worse they tend to feel. The therapeutic goal is not to obliterate the intrusive imagery, but to contain it. Just as with intrusive thoughts in OCD (*see* Chapter 8), *thought-stopping strategies* can be useful. The patient can be instructed to place an elastic band on their wrist and every time the intrusion occurs, to pull the elastic band and let it go (this is a simplified version of aversion therapy). Simultaneously, they tell themselves they will watch a 'mental film' of the trauma, for a set period at a certain time of day. Another strategy is for the patient to mentally interrupt their intrusive thoughts when they occur by saying 'stop!' to themselves. Again they can make a mental note to themselves to watch the 'film' of the trauma at a prearranged time. This leaves more of the patient's day free from intrusions. When the time comes to watch the 'mental film' later on, many patients no longer feel the need.

The above simple strategies generate within the patient a sense of mastery over the intrusions, rather than feeling controlled by them.

Desensitisation. When intrusions persist despite containment strategies, desensitisation techniques may be successful. Desensitisation effectively increases a patient's distress and feeling of lack of control before reducing it, and so should only be employed when a sound therapeutic alliance has been developed and the patient has a good understanding of what is involved.

The procedure involves repeated exposure to thoughts, imagery and feelings associated with the trauma in order for habituation to occur. This can be done verbally in sessions with a therapist, into a tape recorder, which patients can play back to themselves, or by writing out an account of the event which they can read to themselves. The patient should use one of these methods to re-experience the trauma on a daily basis, and only stop thinking about the events once their distress levels have reduced. Relaxation and breathing techniques can be employed during desensitisation to enable the patient to keep control of the amount of fear to which they are exposed. Ideally, for habituation to occur, the patient will need to expose themselves to an intermediate level of fear and to remain 'engaged' until their distress levels reduce.

Cognitive restructuring. This strategy involves enabling the patient to represent the 'whole picture' of the trauma and not use a mental filter to ignore any positive aspects. The purpose of cognitive restructuring for PTSD is for the patient to describe and have a correct mental picture of the trauma as it actually was. This can be helped by identifying the specific thoughts or self-statements related to the trauma that generate distress, then modifying negative statements, replacing them with positive and more balanced thoughts.

Balancing out. Major traumas tend to leave very graphic and vivid impressions in the patient's memory. With PTSD any memories of positive events in the patient's past life become less available, accessible and vivid. Therefore, trauma memories assume an overwhelming importance in the patient's emotional state and their view of the world. In this case, enabling them to access positive memories and use them to counterbalance negative ones proves to be a worthwhile therapeutic task. The therapist aims to reverse the tendency to remember generality rather than specifics by encouraging depth and vividness of the positive memories listed by the patient.

Avoidance reactions

Patients may avoid situations that stimulate recollection of the trauma, and also attempt to escape situations they perceive to be similar to the trauma. They often become hypervigilant to their surroundings and overly sensitive to a sense of danger or threat. Avoidance behaviour generalises well beyond the context of the original trauma and can result in a circumscribed lifestyle, with decreased activity and opportunity for pleasure or achievement.

Desensitisation to avoided situations. As with situations avoided due to any anxiety disorder, desensitisation and graded exposure are the most powerful techniques to employ. A graded hierarchy (or fear ladder, *see* Chapters 3 and 4) should be constructed incorporating all the situations avoided, from the least to the most difficult. Homework assignments involve exposure, first by imagining the situation and then progressing to entering real-life situations, where practical.

Reassessing the degree of threat. Where patients avoid situations because they believe themselves to be in danger or under threat, cognitive restructuring is employed to realistically reassess the danger they are facing. This incorporates the correcting of cognitive biases as listed in Box 7.9.

Each time the patient thinks about the trauma, they can be instructed to check through this list to identify any cognitive biases influencing their interpretation of the event. The therapist can also challenge their beliefs at two levels: inference and evaluation. Inferential questions seek to ascertain whether something is actually true, helping them to view things more realistically, weighing up the evidence for and against that thought/belief. Evaluative questions often consist of 'So what if that were true? What would be so important/awful about that?'. This 'downward arrow' technique is used to elucidate the patient's 'bottom-line belief', their core assumption about the world.

Box 7.9 Cognitive biases in environmental appraisal

- *All or nothing thinking* – everything is seen in black and white terms, e.g. 'I am either in complete control of what is happening or I am not'
- *Overgeneralisation* – expecting a uniform response from people because of the actions of one, e.g. 'All men are potential rapists'
- *Mental filter* – seizing on a negative fragment of a situation and dwelling on it, e.g. 'I could have been killed'
- *Automatic discounting* – ignoring positive aspects of what was achieved despite the trauma, e.g. 'I was only doing my duty in saving the child'
- *Jumping to conclusions* – assuming you know what others are thinking, e.g. 'They all think I should be over it by now, it was 6 weeks ago after all'
- *Magnification and minimisation* – magnifying shortcomings and minimising strengths, e.g. 'Since the trauma I am so irritable with the family and only just about manage to keep working'
- *Emotional reasoning* – focusing on emotional state to draw conclusions about oneself, e.g. 'Since it happened, I'm so jumpy, I guess I'm just a wimp'
- *'Should' statements* – inappropriate use of moral imperatives, should, must, have, ought, e.g. 'It's ridiculous that since the attack I now have to take my daughter shopping with me. I should be able to go by myself'
- *Labelling and mislabelling* – e.g. 'I used to think of myself as a strong person. I could handle anything, but now I'm just weak'
- *Personalisation* – assuming responsibility for things going wrong, e.g. 'I keep thinking over how I handled that situation. I must have made a mistake for the child to have died'

From Scott and Stradling (1995).

Task orientation and problem solving. A practical problem-solving approach can be used to enable the patient to re-engage in routine and community activities, whilst encouraging task orientation to focus on their hassles sequentially. The procedure involved in problem solving is discussed in greater detail in Chapter 9, along with a patient sheet.

CBT treatment approaches

Psychological treatment for PTSD mainly encompasses a cognitive-behaviour approach, in an attempt to address the cardinal symptoms of the disorder.

The basic techniques employed in CBT of other anxiety-related disorders, as described throughout this text, can also be applied to the anxiety provoked by re-experiencing phenomena and to overcome avoidance associated with trauma stimuli. The basic tenets remain the same, however, workers in the field have divergent opinions as to whether it is more effective to focus on the traumatic event itself, or to pay attention mainly to developing coping skills to enable the patient to continue with everyday life. Commonly, in such discussions, the middle line is usually the most popular, recommending a combination of the two approaches and avoiding an extremist position.

In recent years however, there has been greater interest amongst clinicians and researchers regarding PTSD and its treatment. This is thought to reflect the increasing recognition of the disorder. Several new therapeutic techniques have been developed, based upon the eradication of visual memories associated with the trauma. These empirical visualising techniques will be briefly discussed following a description of the more widely used and conventional cognitive-behaviour methods. There now follows a description of four different treatment packages developed specifically for PTSD.

Stress inoculation training (SIT)

Based on Meichenbaum's (1985) approach, SIT is aimed at giving the patient a sense of mastery over their fears by teaching a variety of basic CBT coping skills adapted to their own particular needs. The skills are taught in sessions with the therapist, practiced at home until proficiency is reached and then applied to a graded hierarchy of stresses. Once mastery of these skills has been achieved with everyday stresses, the trauma-related target behaviours are confronted, in sequence.

SIT has been adapted for use with women who have suffered rape, with a successful outcome (Kilpatrick et al., 1982). The techniques have been employed in both individual and group settings. Box 7.10 describes the skills taught in SIT, applied to the three factors involved in the maintenance of anxiety: physiological, behavioural and cognitive.

Box 7.10   Coping skills taught in SIT

Physiological:

- Relaxation — progressive muscular relaxation (*see* Chapter 9 for instructions)

- Breath control — deep diaphragmatic breathing

Behavioural:

- Covert modelling — the patient visualises a fear- or anxiety-provoking situation and imagines themselves coping with it successfully. The patient is encouraged to focus on current situations avoided due to trauma, rather than the past traumatic event itself

- Role-playing — patient and therapist act out successful coping in anxiety-producing scenes with which the patient expects to be confronted

Cognitive:

- Thought stopping — patient generates ruminative thought patterns about the feared stimulus, which are interrupted, initially by the therapist shouting the word 'stop!' and clapping their hands loudly
 — patient learns to use 'stop!' subvocally or devise their own covert thought-stopping term or visualisation

- Guided self-dialogue — patient learns to focus on their own internal thought processes and identify negative irrational or maladaptive self-statements
 — they practice substituting more adaptive self-vocalisations, realistically assessing the probability of danger, controlling self-criticism/devaluation and finally self-praise for their effort

Prolonged exposure

This adaptation of a CBT approach is based on the emotional processing model of fear, proposing that PTSD results from inadequate processing of the trauma stimuli, responses to the trauma and the meaning associated with them.

Treatment requires activation of the fear memory through exposure techniques. The patient is encouraged to describe the traumatic event in detail and is helped to process the memories until they are no longer intensely painful. Over subsequent sessions, the patient is encouraged to include more and more detail about both external and internal cues, such as thoughts, physiological responses and feared consequences. Descriptions are repeated several times each session and care is taken to ensure anxiety levels decrease before the session is terminated.

As with CBT for other anxiety-related disorders, exposure is most successful when combined with reciprocal inhibition (incompatible behaviours and thoughts, such as muscular relaxation and coping thoughts) and systematic desensitisation to avoided stimuli by the use of a graded hierarchy. The hierarchy can include thoughts or images related to the trauma, as well as everyday activities avoided due to fear of further danger and thoughts of vulnerability. The cognitive changes associated with such behavioural tests can be monitored by the use of thought diaries as described elsewhere in this text (*see* Chapter 3, Figure 3.6).

Cognitive processing therapy (CPT)

This is a therapy model developed to treat the specific symptoms of PTSD in victims of sexual assault (Resick and Schnicke, 1992), based on the information-processing model of PTSD. It combines the main tenets of exposure therapies with cognitive restructuring. The cognitive component of therapy challenges specific cognitions most likely to have been disrupted as a result of the trauma.

Systematic exposure to traumatic memory in a safe environment is helpful in the re-evaluation of threat-cues and habituation to them. However, victims may still blame themselves and feel shame, disgust and anger to a sufficiently intense degree to generate intrusive memories, heightened arousal and avoidance reactions. CPT aims to activate traumatic memories whilst simultaneously providing corrective information for faulty attributions or expectations to enable complete processing of the trauma. The trauma encountered generates new information about the self and the world that is in conflict with previously held cognitive schemas. These conflicts may be concerned with danger and safety ('I don't feel safe going out alone') but also include other themes such as self-esteem, body-image, competence and intimacy. CPT focuses on identifying and resolving 'stuck points', i.e. conflicts between prior schemas and new information. The four main core assumptions which are thought to be violated by trauma are:

- the world is a safe place (invulnerability)
- a sense of self-worth
- other people can be trusted
- the world is a meaningful place.

The overwhelming emotional experience observed in PTSD is thought to arise from the mismatch between the person's view of the world, based on the aforementioned core assumptions, and new information about the world as a result of the trauma. When this new information is not easily integrated into his/her existing model of the world, then PTSD symptoms appear. The process of cognitive integration is reflected in the oscillation between intrusive experiences and denial with emotional numbing.

The exposure component consists of patients writing about the event in detail including sensory memories, thoughts and feelings during the event. They are instructed to read this account to themselves daily; in sessions the therapist helps them label their feelings and resolve 'stuck points'.

Eye movement desensitisation treatment

Eye movement desensitisation and reprocessing (EMDR) has been applied to the treatment of PTSD. Despite the lack of a convincing theoretical basis to explain its effect, there is growing clinical evidence of its efficacy. It was first described by Shapiro (1989) and thus far has been viewed as a purely empirical treatment. The procedure is relatively complex, but basically consists of the patient performing repetitive rapid eye movements whilst imagining the traumatic event in their 'mind's eye'. Treatment is focused upon visual memories of the most traumatic point of the event, salient personal meanings related to the event and associated physical sensations.

Shapiro demonstrated that EMDR produced a very rapid desensitisation effect on the flashbacks and traumatised memories, so that the trauma event was easily brought into memory but was now unassociated with anxiety or negative affect. Proponents suggest that EMDR usually requires an average of only four sessions (which may be delivered in one day) to extinguish extreme fear reactions, compared with six to eight sessions with conventional exposure therapy.

This relatively new treatment has attracted controversy and despite several controlled trials supporting its effectiveness, doubts remain amongst mental health professionals.

Debriefing

It has become popular to offer debriefing after major national disasters (e.g. following the Lockerbie plane crash), but its efficacy remains questionable. This is because certain large-scale studies (e.g. following large Australian bush fires) have shown that debriefing does not reduce the incidence of stress disorders following such disasters. However, it remains something of a political perogative to provide such a service to victims of large-scale trauma.

Other approaches which show some promise involve a trained counsellor facilitating sessions in 'critical incident stress debriefing'. Large companies (such as high-street building societies) employ such professionals to debrief staff following armed raids. The aim of the group session is to allow and encourage members of the group to 'tell their story', thereby exposing themselves to memories of the trauma. Additional benefits include gaining emotional support from their colleagues and attaining a realistic view of the incident based on all the available information. This approach has yet to be subjected to the rigours of randomised, controlled trials.

Appendix 7A

DSM-IV and ICD-10 criteria for PTSD

Both the ICD-10 and the DSM-IV require the presence of the following symptoms occurring after trauma:

- re-experiencing phenomena

  - recurrent intrusive recollections
  - recurrent distressing dreams
  - acting or feeling as if the event were still occurring
  - distress on exposure to cues that recall the event

- avoidance of associated stimuli

  - avoid activity or places associated with the trauma
  - diminished interest or participation in activities
  - detachment or estrangement from others
  - restricted range of affect (e.g. unable to feel love)

- increased arousal

  - insomnia
  - increased anger
  - poor concentration
  - hypervigilance.

ICD-10 requires that these features manifest within 6 months of cessation of the stressor.

DSM-IV recognises sub-categories of PTSD as follows:

- acute – symptoms last less than 3 months

- chronic – symptoms for more than 3 months

- delayed onset – starting more than 6 months after trauma.

Areas of enquiry for PTSD case assessment

- Motivation
  - Have you had any particular problems since the trauma?
  - Any recurring memories of it that interfere with your enjoyment of life?
  - Do you want help for any problems that have arisen?
  - Do you feel others have pushed you into seeking help?

- Traumatic event
  - When did it happen?
  - What kind of memories interfere with your enjoyment of life?
  - What happened to you exactly?
  - Did you think you were going to die?
  - Were you injured?
  - How do you feel you coped at the time?

- Coping since
  - How do you feel you have coped since the trauma?
  - How have you coped with the unpleasant memories?
  - Do you feel less able to cope with certain situations now?
  - Have you felt so distressed that you've been unable to carry on with the usual things you did before the trauma?

- Avoidance
  - Are there any situations you now avoid?
  - Do you try to avoid thoughts or images related to the trauma?
  - If so, how?

- Intrusions
  - Do you have nightmares about the trauma or similar themes?
  - Do they wake you?
  - Do you recall the details of nightmares on waking?
  - Do you have any intrusive memories (or flashbacks) of the event when you are awake?

	– Is this
	(a) so bad you can't think of or do anything else
	(b) always at the back of your mind but you can carry on
	(c) there occasionally, but it doesn't really bother you?
• Reactivation of earlier trauma	– Has the trauma reawakened any earlier painful memories?
	– Do these trigger any other painful memories?
• Irritability	– Do you find you are more irritable than before the trauma?
	– Do you 'fly off the handle' more than before?
	– Is your irritability linked to present circumstances?
• Symptoms of stress	– Do have frequent headaches?
	– Is your appetite poor?
	– Do you sleep badly?
	– Are you easily fatigued?
	– Are you easily frightened?
	– Do your hands shake?
	– Do you feel nervous, tense or worried?
	– Is your digestion poor?
	– Do you have trouble thinking clearly?
	– Do you feel unhappy?
	– Do you cry more than usual?
	– Do you find it hard to enjoy 'pleasant' activities?
	– Do you find it difficult to make decisions?
	– Is your daily work suffering?
	– Have you lost interest in things?
	– Do you feel worthless?
	– Has the thought of ending your life been in your mind?

• Substance abuse	– Do you use alcohol or drugs to help cope with distress?
	– Do you feel alcohol/drugs are a problem for you?
	– Do those close to you say that the alcohol/drugs you use are a problem to them?
• Impact of event	– Looking at the overall effect the trauma has had on your life, do you think most people would regard it as having been
	(a) not stressful
	(b) mildly so
	(c) moderately
	(d) severely
	(e) extremely?
	– If (d) or (e) probe why
• Life before trauma	– How satisfied with life were you a year before the trauma?
	– Has the trauma made worse any previous difficulties?
	– Have you had previous trouble with your nerves? (probe)
• Suicidal ideation	– Have you felt life is not worth living?
	– Have you thought of ending your life?
	– Have you made plans to end your life?
	– Have you started to do things according to that plan?
	– Have you actually made an attempt on your life?

Adapted from Scott and Stradling (1995).

8
Obsessive-compulsive disorder

Introduction

Obsessive-compulsive disorder (OCD) is now recognised as a relatively common mental illness with a 6-month prevalence of around 1–2% in the population (Bebbington, 1998). It has been called the 'hidden disease' on account of the deceptiveness with which an apparently benign condition can obscure the real distress and morbidity that can pervade the lives of patients and entire families. Moreover, what was previously seen as primarily a 'neurotic' condition is now increasingly recognised as a neuropsychiatric disorder involving abnormalities of brain function.

OCD is characterised by recurrent intrusive and senseless thoughts or images (obsessions) leading to repeated behaviours (compulsions). Obsessions are recognised as arising from within the subject's own mind, and are acknowledged by the individual as absurd and pointless; compulsions are 'behaviours' resulting from obsessions, and may be motor acts (such as cleaning) or cognitive acts (such as counting).

Typically, sufferers experience a recurrent and distressing urge to perform a pointless task, although the activity may in some cases have some symbolic significance (e.g. a compulsion may be interpreted by the individual as making restitution for a perceived misdemeanor). The individual characteristically attempts to resist the senseless urge, but this only leads to mounting tension and distress, which is normally only relieved by performing the act, which then becomes ritualised. However, the subsequent reduction in anxiety is only partial and shortlived, and the overwhelming urge to repeat the ritual soon returns. Thus a perpetual cycle is established which may come to dominate the individual's work and home life, the rituals often taking up several hours of each day. Box 8.1 outlines a case history of OCD, emphasising the patient's experience and the consequences of the illness on those around him.

Box 8.1   Case history of OCD

Mr A was a retired office worker with an 18-year history of OCD. Whenever he was introduced to someone and told their name he felt compelled to count in his head to a hundred. Resisting this urge caused such intense anxiety that further conversation was impossible, resulting in misunderstanding and embarrassment. Over the years Mr A had found he no longer resisted the urge to count to a hundred on meeting new people, but the awkwardness created by this ritual led to increasing social withdrawal. Whilst he still enjoyed spending time with his family and grandchildren, his inability to conduct the simplest of business interactions led to sharp arguments with his wife, and it was this that led to him seeing the family doctor.

Aetiology

Genes

Despite ample evidence for a biological substrate to OCD, genetic studies remain inconclusive and difficult to interpret. Nevertheless, twin studies have shown monozygotic concordance for the disorder to be between 53% and 87%. In addition, OCD sufferers have been shown to have a much greater family history of psychiatric illness compared with controls. Moreover, the links between OCD and Gilles de la Tourette's syndrome (GTS – a disorder marked by irrepressible tics and vocalisations) are well recognised, and GTS has an established genetic basis.

Neurobiology

What was once considered to be idiopathic OCD has in fact been shown to be related largely to neuropsychiatric causes. 'Idiopathic' OCD most commonly follows from head injury, birth injury and also focal epilepsy of the temporal lobe. OCD is also seen in Parkinson's disease and Sydenham's chorea (non-choreiform rheumatic fever does not lead to obsessive symptoms), which implies involvement of the basal ganglia, in particular the striatum. Moreover, neuroimaging studies have predominantly found increased activity in the orbitofrontal cortex, caudate nucleus, thalamus and anterior cingulate gyrus. For readers with a special interest in brain function, the current neurobiological theory of OCD is shown graphically in Figure 8.1 below.

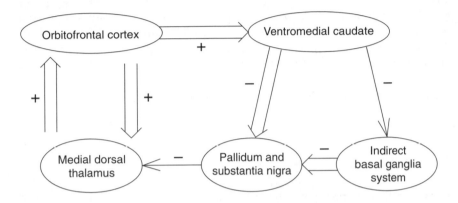

Figure 8.1 The neurobiology of OCD (adapted from Saxena *et al.*, 1998).

The positive feedback between cortex and thalamus, shown on the left of Figure 8.1, is, in normal circumstances, adequately inhibited by input from the globus pallidus and substantia nigra.

This inhibition appears to be lost in OCD owing to inhibition of the striatum itself by direct input from the caudate (top right) and indirectly by other subcortical structures (bottom right). The proposed deficit in striatal suppression of the thalamo-cortical loop results in the inability to neurally 'switch off' obsessions and compulsions generated in this area of the brain.

Neurochemistry

The efficacy of clomipramine (a predominantly serotonergic tricyclic) and SSRIs in the treatment of OCD has emphasised the likely role of serotonin (5-HT, hydroxytryptophan) in the pathogenesis of this disorder. Serotonergic nerve fibres arise in the raphe nuclei of the brainstem and ramify widely throughout the brain, acting as a neural 'pacemaker', regulating the rhythms and homeostasis of the brain. It is thought that a deficiency in this serotonergic brain-regulating mechanism may unmask the clinical features of OCD.

Psychological models

Psychoanalytic

The psychoanalytic theory of Freud proposed that obsessions represent psychological defences against unacceptable unconscious impulses. According to this theory individuals may become fixated at the anal stage of psychosexual development, a stage often marked by conflict with parents; an infant's only form of control is to withold faeces. 'Anally fixated' subjects may go on to repress hostile impulses against their parents by means of obsessive-compulsive behaviours.

Behavioural

Learning theory proposes that OCD arises from an initial experience associated with marked distress, such as losing a loved one as a result of a contagious disease. Using this example, distress then becomes associated with the idea of contagion, and this anxiety is reduced by the act of thorough cleansing after coming into contact with, or even thinking about, dirt. The reduced anxiety associated with cleaning only serves to reinforce the act in the face of further concerns about contagion. Avoidance of situations triggering obsessional thoughts also occurs and, where extensive, can resemble the avoidance behaviours seen in agoraphobia.

Avoidance behaviours prevent, and compulsive behaviours terminate, exposure to the feared stimuli or obsessional thought, producing short-term relief of anxiety but preventing exposure and extinction of anxiety in the long-term. Both avoidance and compulsions prevent the patient from confronting (being exposed to) his fears. These behaviours thus prevent reappraisal: if the patient stops them (response prevention), they discover that the things they are afraid of do not actually happen.

Cognitive

The model recently put forward by cognitive therapists to understand OCD is based on the observation that the very individuals who become extremely distressed by obsessional thoughts relating to harming others or themselves are the people most unlikely to do so. Such individuals have been described as being 'of tender conscience' (Rachman and Hodgson, 1980), excessively conscientious, with high moral or religious standards. They are therefore especially sensitive to intrusive thoughts which impinge upon their strict moral beliefs and are likely to feel obliged to bring restitution for any harm done, albeit imagined. They feel intensely **responsible** for their irrational obsessional impulses to harm others, and thus experience **guilt** that is only assuaged by the penalty of neutralising behaviours which develop into obsessional disorders. Neutralising behaviour consists of actions or thoughts which the individual considers 'put right' the obsession; they are also termed 'compulsions' and tend to be stereotyped, often becoming ritualised.

The distress consequent to thinking a thought such as 'I might pick up that knife and stab my child with it' is really provoked by the person's **appraisal** of that thought – that 'I must be a really bad mother to even think such an awful thing!'. Salkovskis (1988) proposes that 'obsessional thoughts' and intrusions are a natural, normal phenomenon to which we usually pay no attention whatsoever. However, vulnerable individuals become very distressed and shocked by such 'normal' thoughts, insisting that they are completely out of character and becoming acutely aware of their occurrence. Also, mood disturbance is implicated in that depression is seen as reducing an individual's natural barrier to noticing such fleeting thoughts and serves to bias access to negative self-appraisals. A cognitive-behaviour model of OCD is illustrated in Figure 8.2.

This model helps explain why receiving reassurance and the sharing of responsibility are so powerful in protecting the individual from distress associated with obsessional thoughts; if something awful were then to happen, they would not be wholly responsible for it. The seeking of reassurance or the presence of a 'responsibility figure' (i.e. the therapist or doctor) are similar to neutralising behaviours or avoidance in that they prevent the patient being exposed to the distressing thoughts.

Treatment is focused on: the identified maintaining factors; reducing avoidance behaviour and increasing exposure to problem situations and thoughts; the modification of attitudes concerning personal responsibility; modification of their appraisal of their intrusive thoughts; on preventing neutralising, which follows both the appraisal of intrusive thoughts and the appraisal of responsibility; and increasing exposure to responsibility, by direct exposure and stopping reassurance seeking.

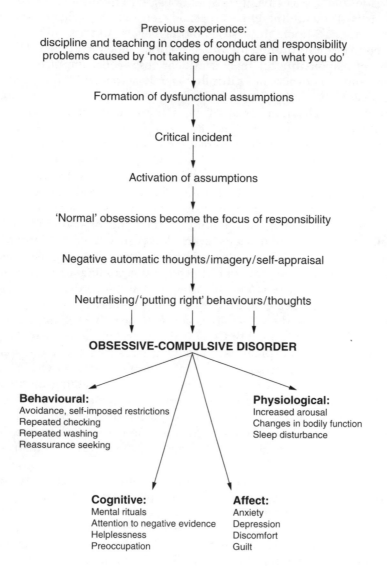

Previous experience:
discipline and teaching in codes of conduct and responsibility
problems caused by 'not taking enough care in what you do'

↓

Formation of dysfunctional assumptions

↓

Critical incident

↓

Activation of assumptions

↓

'Normal' obsessions become the focus of responsibility

↓

Negative automatic thoughts/imagery/self-appraisal

↓

Neutralising/'putting right' behaviours/thoughts

↓ ↓ ↓

OBSESSIVE-COMPULSIVE DISORDER

Behavioural:
Avoidance, self-imposed restrictions
Repeated checking
Repeated washing
Reassurance seeking

Physiological:
Increased arousal
Changes in bodily function
Sleep disturbance

Cognitive:
Mental rituals
Attention to negative evidence
Helplessness
Preoccupation

Affect:
Anxiety
Depression
Discomfort
Guilt

Figure 8.2 Cognitive-behaviour model: development of OCD (after Salkovskis and Warwick, 1988).

Clinical features

Obsessive-compulsive symptoms tend to cluster in a few well-recognised categories: checking rituals, cleaning rituals, obsessive thoughts and obsessional slowness; some show mixed rituals and a small, but important, group self-harm by cutting themselves. The management of the latter is typically the premise of highly specialised services, and will not be considered in this chapter. Box 8.2 lists the common obsessional thoughts with associated compulsions.

Cleaning rituals

People with cleaning rituals may feel compelled to wash themselves repeatedly or clean household surfaces again and again after coming into contact with essentially harmless, if non-sterile, objects. These cleaning rituals may take up much of the day, leaving the individual in a state of exhaustion, and not infrequently result in physical complications such as dermatitis. The anxiety provoked by thoughts of uncleanliness can lead to demands on members of the family to participate in rituals, or at least to keep away from cleaned surfaces and the like. Sufferers are often embarrassed to disclose their fruitless rituals, knowing that they seem senseless (to themselves and others), and for this reason presentation may be delayed until either the patient becomes unable to function in their activities of daily living, or relationships begin to suffer. The incessant and pointless cycle of obsessions and compulsions commonly leads to depression, and consequently a proportion of patients with OCD may present with symptoms of a depressive illness.

Checking rituals

People with checking rituals may have experienced a triggering event such as a burglary or housefire, either in their own homes or those of friends or relatives. The sufferer becomes unduly anxious at the thought of leaving a door unlocked or a cooker switched on, and as a result goes throughout the house checking locks or switches (or both). Thus, the individual may find themselves delayed for work in the morning on account of checking the house repeatedly for security, and at night may be unable to get to bed until hours of repeated checking that power sockets are switched off and electric plugs removed. The family may

Box 8.2 Common obsessions and associated compulsive behaviours

Obsession	Compulsion
1 Contamination (ideas of being harmed by contact with substances believed to be dangerous, e.g. dirt, germs, urine, faeces, blood, radiation, poison, etc.)	
'The hairdresser's comb had AIDS'	Ring doctor; check body for symptoms; virus on it; wash hands and hair; sterilise objects
2 Physical violence to self or others, by self or others	
'I will harm my baby'	Won't be left alone with the baby; seeks reassurance; hides knives, plastic bags
3 Death	
Images of loved ones dead	Imagines the same people alive
4 Accidental harm (e.g. accident, illness)	
'I may have hit someone with my car'	Telephone hospitals, police; retraces route driven; checks car for marks
5 Socially unacceptable behaviour (e.g. shouting, swearing, losing control)	
'I am going to shout an obscenity'	Tries to 'keep control of behaviour'; avoids social situations; asks for reassurance that behaviour is acceptable
6 Sex (preoccupation with sexual organs, unacceptable acts)	
'I am going to rape someone'	Avoids being alone with women; tries to keep mind off sexual thoughts
7 Religion (e.g. blasphemous thoughts, religious doubts)	
'I am going to offer my food to the devil''	Prays; seeks religious help/confession; offers other things to God
8 Orderliness (things being in the right place, actions done in the right way, according to a particular pattern or number)	
'If I don't clean my teeth in the right way, I'll have to do it again until I get it right''	Repeats action a 'good' number of times; repeats until it 'feels right'
9 Nonsense (meaningless phrases, images, tunes, strings of numbers, words)	
Hears (in head) tune of a TV sports programme while reading	Repeats action until manages to read the same passage without the tune occurring

unwittingly reinforce these compulsive behaviours by colluding in rituals in order to avoid the unacceptable levels of distress in the subject that can cause much conflict. As with other obsessive-compulsive behaviours, those with checking rituals may present late with deterioration in social or work function, or with depression.

Obsessive thoughts

Individuals suffering with obssessive thoughts may be plagued by the thought of doing something grossly unacceptable and alienating, and it is recognised that such people are usually the least likely to act on these urges. Hence, a fastidious and caring mother may be subject to recurrent unwanted thoughts of stabbing her child, and as a result does not allow the child into the kitchen where the knives are kept. Another example is that of a man plagued by thoughts that he may inappropriately touch female colleagues at work, causing him to avoid being alone in the same room as them. In cases of obssessive thoughts, presentation to the doctor again usually follows the disruption of work or social functioning, or the development of depressive symptoms.

Obsessional slowness

In obsessional slowness the subject may be obsessed with the quality of workmanship in ordinary tasks like cleaning a car or decorating a room. As a result of the self-imposed standards of perfection, procedures become painstakingly slow to the extent that even the simplest tasks take an inordinately long time to complete, and many routine household endeavours may ultimately remain uncompleted due to the excessive slowness with which they are performed. For example, a man suffering with obsessional slowness may find he has spent an entire weekend attempting to paint a windowsill in the house, never getting beyond sanding down the old paint because he never achieves the regular surface he feels is necessary. Subsequent weekends give rise to other little household jobs, few of which are ever completed, and the marriage relationship may suffer as a result. Typically, it is either the effect of the illness on others, or supervening depression, which eventually leads to consultation with a doctor.

Diagnosis of OCD

The diagnosis of primary OCD is usually straightforward, reflecting the easily recognised and characterisitic features of obsessions and compulsions outlined above. Occasionally a patient may present with depressive symptoms, and as 20% of people with depression have a marked obsessive-compulsive component to their illness, it is advisable always to ask about symptoms of OCD in patients presenting as depressed. It is important when interviewing these patients to be sensitive to the real and intense distress that symptoms of OCD produce, even where the thoughts or acts disclosed seem quite bizarre or even frankly amusing.

The diagnostic criteria for OCD are given in ICD-10, as shown in the Appendix to this chapter, together with the diagnostic criteria for OCD given in DSM-IV.

Differential diagnosis of OCD

Primary OCD is usually not problematic to diagnose. However, as has been discussed already, OCD may present following, or in the context of, a number of other disorders. In particular, obsessive-compulsive features have been noted in pervasive developmental disorders of childhood (notably autism and Asperger's syndrome), as well as in anankastic (obsessional) personality disorder, temporal lobe epilepsy and schizophrenia. OCD is also commonly seen in depression, after head injuries and following the onset of idiopathic Parkinson's disease. Strict adherence to systematic enquiry will usually avail correct clinical diagnosis, although some cases remain hard to differentiate even with adequate background information (for example, high-functioning autism, schizotypal illness/personality and OCD). The differential diagnosis of OCD is summarised in Box 8.3.

Anorexia nervosa and OCD

It is interesting to note that links between OCD and anorexia nervosa have been observed for many years, and obsessive-compulsive traits have been identified in up to 80% of people with anorexia. Those suffering with anorexia can be said to have obsessions and compulsions relating to food and body image (although these are not resisted, and

Box 8.3   The differential diagnosis of OCD

- primary depression
- phobic illness (e.g. social)
- anankastic personality
- autism and Asperger's syndrome
- temporal lobe epilepsy
- Tourette's syndrome
- schizophrenia

abnormal body image is traditionally termed an over-valued idea and the resulting behaviours make sense to the individual). Moreover, these individuals not infrequently present with coexisting symptoms that *are* characteristic of OCD, and these deserve treatment in their own right. Where anorexia *is* suspected it should be vigorously assessed and treated (the appropriate management of anorexia is discussed in a separate text).

Assessment of OCD

The assessment of OCD is usually straightforward, insofar as patients seeking help tend to recognise and volunteer their symptoms. However, where the compulsions are perceived to be unacceptable (e.g. bizarre sexual urges) then clearly a very sympathetic interviewing style is required. The differential diagnosis should always be borne in mind, including possible organic causes such as stroke. The important features of assessment are summarised in Box 8.4.

Treatment of OCD

Pharmacotherapy

The treatment of OCD has traditionally been predominantly psychological, reflecting both the widely held view of the illness as a psychological disorder, and the limited drugs available for its treatment. However, it has been observed since the 1960s that obsessive-compulsive

---

Box 8.4   Assessment of OCD

- Twenty per cent of people with depression have a marked obsessive-compulsive component to their illness, therefore it is advisable always to ask about symptoms of OCD in patients presenting as depressed.

- A significant proportion of patients with OCD become depressed as a result, and it is therefore advisable to ask about symptoms of depression in those presenting with 'primary' OCD.

- Ask about the separate aspects of checking, cleaning, slowness or obsessive thoughts and ascertain their perceived meaning to the individual.

- Ask about the level of distress caused, and any effects on relationships. Is the family involved in the rituals in any way?

- Specifically ask about the effects the symptoms are having on daily functioning, including work and social life.

- If there is marked distress, ask about suicidal thoughts. OCD is a known risk factor in completed suicide.

---

behaviour frequently responds to drugs with marked serotonergic activity, in particular clomipramine (a tricyclic antidepressant). More recently, SSRIs have been used with benefit in the treatment of OCD. Those SSRIs currently licensed for the treatment of OCD are sertraline, fluoxetine, fluvoxamine and paroxetine, as well as clomipramine, and these are shown in Box 8.5.

In prescribing medication for OCD it should be recognised that drug therapy alone is unlikely to effect a long-term cure, and where services allow, it should be given in conjunction with psychological intervention as described later in this chapter. SSRIs are the drug of first choice, as they are less toxic in terms of side-effects and overdose, but clomipramine remains valuable in those cases where there has been a previous good response, or where there is no response to SSRIs.

Psychological treatment

The principles of treatment are derived from the psychological models outlined earlier. The traditional approach to OCD has been behavioural,

---

Box 8.5   Drug treatment of OCD

Sertraline: 50 mg daily increasing gradually, if necessary, to a max. of 200 mg OD

Fluoxetine: 20 mg daily increasing gradually, if necessary, to a max. of 60 mg OD

Fluvoxamine: 100 mg daily increasing gradually, if necessary, to a max. of 300 mg OD

Paroxetine: 20 mg daily increasing gradually, if necessary, to a max. of 60 mg OD

Clomipramine: 10 mg daily increasing gradually, if necessary, to a max. of 250 mg OD

Maintenance dose should continue for 3–6 months after remission of symptoms, to reduce the risk of relapse.

---

comprising **exposure** to the distressing thoughts with **response prevention**, i.e. not responding to the obsessions with ritualistic, compulsive behaviours or thoughts. Recently, workers in the field have established the use of cognitive aspects in treatment, as well as in the understanding and conceptualising of OCD (Salkovskis, 1985, 1988; Rachman, 1993). Clearly, the time required for appropriate explanation and application of the psychological treatment of OCD is far greater than the GP has available. Owing to this and the often chronic and difficult nature of OCD, the majority of patients are best treated by experienced cognitive-behaviour therapists. However, interested GPs will find the following aspects of treatment useful and may wish to undertake treatment alongside community mental health nurse input. Specialist referral should be considered for particularly severe or chronic OCD, or in the absence of improvement. Box 8.6 illustrates difficulties commonly encountered in the assessment and treatment of patients with OCD.

Behavioural aspects

Following from the behavioural model of OCD, treatment involves exposing people to the feared stimuli (including distressing thoughts and previously avoided situations), while encouraging them to block any behaviours which prevent or terminate this exposure. Patients are told that they will eventually be expected to confront the anxiety brought on by a distressing thought 'without switching it off by the

---

Box 8.6 Difficulties in assessment and treatment of OCD

- Chronicity
  - compulsive behaviour and avoidance so extensive that the patient is no longer aware of the preceding pattern of obsessive thoughts

- Patient reluctant to discuss thoughts
  - they feel the content of the thoughts are unacceptable and repugnant
  - they think the therapist will think them unpleasant and may reject them
  - they fear that talking about their obsessions makes them real and thereby more powerful
  - as insight into the irrationality of thoughts and behaviours is retained, patients find them socially embarrassing and shameful
  - they fear the therapist may take action against them due to their thoughts, e.g. a mother with thoughts of harming her children fears social services involvement

---

rituals', that the best way to deal with the thoughts is to 'get used to them'; they then discover that the things they are most afraid of do not actually happen. They will be shown and taught ways to deal with the distress and to stop the thoughts causing the distress. A fear hierarchy, similar to that used with patients with phobias or panic (*see* Chapters 4 and 5), is used to identify situations suitable for graded exposure, be they situations previously avoided or where neutralising behaviours are employed. As with any graded exposure programme, the exposure can be modelled, imagined or *in vivo*. Relaxation can be learnt and employed in the distressing situations to aid response prevention (*see* Chapter 9). Patients should use recording sheets to plan and rate their achievements, in order to monitor their own progress (*see* Figure 8.3 for an example of a suitable recording sheet).

Behavioural experiments with the therapist, provoking a situation they would normally avoid and not make any attempts to reduce their anxiety, will show the patient that although their anxiety reaches a peak, it will reduce with time in the absence of the rituals. Some patients will not be able to attempt this initially, in which case they can observe the

Date and time	Situation and general feeling	Distressing thoughts	Anxiety level 0–100	Checking/rituals – actions or thoughts	How long did it last? How many times?	Did you manage to stop? How?	Who else involved in checking?

Figure 8.3 Monitoring sheet for checking compulsions.

therapist modelling the situation to them (e.g. the therapist touching the sole of their shoe or a toilet seat). Often the time required for anxiety levels to normalise in such sessions may stretch to 2 hours; clearly well outside the time available to GPs for an individual patient. It may therefore be useful to recruit the help of a 'psychologically minded' relative or a community mental health nurse to remain with the patient and prevent any compulsive behaviours. Family members who may be inadvertently reinforcing avoidance of responsibility by agreeing to carry out rituals themselves should be encouraged to stop, if necessary telling the patient 'It is the doctor's orders that I don't do this.'

'**Thought stopping**' is a simple, yet effective, means of blocking obsessional thoughts, thereby alleviating discomfort and leading to a reduction in compulsive behaviour. It is also of use in the treatment of PTSD (*see* Chapter 7). As it is a 'self-help' strategy, it serves to increase the patient's sense of control over their own problem. The patient is told to focus on an obsessional thought and then say 'stop!' to themselves. This is followed by focusing on a pre-planned, alternative pattern of thoughts which the patient has chosen to be pleasant and relaxing. Clearly, this procedure requires practice with the therapist prior to applying it to a range of obsessional thoughts. Practice usually begins with the patient talking themselves through the procedure (overt practice), before applying it silently in their mental thoughts (covert practice). Once this process is learnt, the patient enters previously avoided situations to provoke obsessional thoughts in order to apply thought stopping.

The aim of behavioural treatment is to teach the patient skills and strategies which they can apply for themselves in any future situations. Therefore, it is imperative that the rationale for treatment is clearly understood and the patients are able to take responsibility for continuing with their own treatment plan, under gradually reducing levels of guidance from the therapist. As in any behaviour therapy, as treatment proceeds, it should become more and more patient directed. Guidelines for 'normal behaviour' (*see* Appendix 8A) can be agreed with the patient and these will help in preventing relapse in the future.

Cognitive aspects

Cognitive techniques are frequently used in combination with the behavioural methods outlined above. In addition to exposure and response prevention, cognitive aspects of treatment focus on changing the beliefs and thoughts which directly cause distress in obsessional patients. Patients are encouraged to modify the negative appraisals of their obsessional thoughts and change their erroneous beliefs about their own responsibility. The usual setting for this is in conducting behavioural experiments. Behavioural tests are set up which focus on the patient's specific fears, e.g. 'If I do that . . . will happen.' and the validity of these fears are thus tested. During planned exposure to their distressing thoughts, patients are encouraged to give a running commentary of their thought pattern. This enables the identification of negative automatic thoughts and appraisals of responsibility. They attempt to answer these with alternative, more accurate thoughts and self-statements.

Neutralising thoughts or behaviours (compulsions) prevent accurate reappraisal of true risks of a certain action and further amplify pre-existing beliefs about responsibility. Therefore, exposure with response prevention in the absence of the feared outcome enables the patient to make a more accurate appraisal of how much their obsessional thoughts really represent threat. In short, they learn that thinking the obsessional thought and doing nothing to set it right does not result in disaster, and allowing themselves to think the thought does not cause it to happen in real life.

The cognitive model of obsessions gives the perception of respons-ibility for harm to self or others a key role. Treatment aims to change the patient's views about responsibility by demonstrating that the taking of previously avoided responsibility does not have dire consequences. This is explained in further detail in Box 8.7.

The issue of reassurance is important in cognitive work with obsessives, as it is a way of spreading the responsibility. It is a form of avoidance from responsibility, similar to getting family members to check after you. The therapist or doctor has to ensure that they do not perpetuate this avoidance by providing the patient with inappropriate

---

Box 8.7   Exposure to responsibility

Exposure to responsibility can be implemented by:

- getting the patient to undertake previously avoided activities involving elements of responsibility, e.g. being the last one to retire for the night
- demonstrating the effects of reassurance-seeking, then prevent-ing the seeking of reassurance
- getting the patient to seek out responsibility actively without revealing any details to friends, family or therapist, so that they alone are responsible

reassurance. The patient has to come to trust in their own judgement of safety and situations without persistent checking, and this will cause them to modify their attitudes concerning responsibility.

Relapse prevention

This is best accomplished once all rituals, both overt (behaviours) and covert (mental activities) have been fully response-prevented during exposure. It is useful to discuss with the patient hypothetical situations which may bring the obsessions back and for them to produce written advice for themselves should a relapse occur. An example of a 'setback sheet' is given in Box 8.8.

Discussion of factors to predict setbacks should include reference to

---

Box 8.8 Patient's 'setback sheet'

- Take things in steps, don't take on something I am not ready to handle
- Tasks that you decide to do should be handled in stages, don't worry if some are not mastered, you will have some 'off days'. Don't give up because one time didn't work out right
- After doing tasks, however distressing, the thing to remember is that anxiety will come down
- Use relaxation techniques to help here
- All thoughts, however distressing, should be taken hold of and analysed, retraining my mind
- Remember the things that help:
  - letting thoughts and anxieties float over you, let them flow straight through your mind
  - answering worrying thoughts so that a crazy, mixed-up thought becomes a more level-headed, reasonable thought, more like reality than fantasy
  - taking control of situations like counting
- Allow myself to feel feelings. It is not wrong to feel or think anything
- Talk to people; don't bottle up feelings and anxieties
- When thoughts come, if you can think them through without acting on them by checking, half the battle's won

stress and anxiety from external sources, depressed mood, extra responsibilities and being tired. Therefore, when a setback occurs, rather than focusing on the content of the distressing thoughts themselves, the patient is able to attribute correctly the distress they are experiencing to their thoughts.

Appendix 8A

ICD-10 diagnostic criteria for OCD

The patient should have obsessions, compulsions or both, which should be present on most days for at least 2 weeks (although most patients will have suffered for considerably longer). The obsessions and compulsions share the following features, all of which should be present:

- they must be acknowledged as originating within the mind and not imposed by outside persons; this distinguishes OCD from schizophrenia

- the obsessions and compulsions must be repetitive and unpleasant, and should be recognised as unreasonable or excessive

- the patient must try to resist the thoughts coming into their mind, and try to resist performing the compulsive act, although in very long-standing illness resistance may be minimal. At least one obsession or compulsion unsuccessfully resisted should be present

- the obsessional thought or compulsion should not be pleasurable in itself, although it may bring temporary relief from anxiety

- the symptom must cause either distress or some kind of interference with social or individual functioning, usually by wasting time.

DSM-IV diagnostic criteria for OCD

Either obsessions or compulsions.
  Obsessions as defined by 1–4:

1 recurrent and persistent thoughts, impulses or images that are experienced at some time as intrusive and inappropriate and that cause marked anxiety or distress;

2 the thoughts, impulses or images are not simply excessive worries about real-life problems;

3 the person attempts to ignore or suppress such thoughts, impulses or images, or to neutralise them with some other thought or action;

4 the person recognises that the thoughts, impulses or images are a product of his or her own mind (not imposed from without as in thought insertion).

Compulsions as defined by 1 and 2:

1 repetitive behaviours (e.g. hand-washing, ordering, checking) or mental acts (counting, repeating words silently) that the person feels driven to perform in response to an obsession, or according to rules that must be applied rigidly;

2 the behaviours are aimed at preventing or reducing distress or averting some dreaded event; however, these acts either are not connected in a realistic way with what they are designed to neutralise, or are clearly excessive.

Guidelines for 'normal behaviour'

Washing:

- do not exceed one 10-minute shower daily
- do not exceed five hand-washings per day, 30 seconds each
- restrict hand-washing to when hands are visibly dirty or sticky
- continue to expose yourself deliberately on a weekly basis to objects or situations that used to disturb you
- if objects or situations are still somewhat disturbing, expose yourself twice weekly to them
- do not avoid situations that cause discomfort. If you detect a tendency to avoid a situation, confront it deliberately at least twice a week

Checking:

- do not check more than once any objects or situations that used to trigger an urge to check
- do not check even once in situations that your therapist has advised you do not require checking
- do not avoid situations that trigger an urge to check. If you detect a tendency to avoid, confront these situations deliberately twice a week and exercise control by not checking
- do not assign responsibility for checking to friends or family members in order to avoid checking

Adapted from Riggs and Foa (1993).

Two sheets for people with obsessive-compulsive problems:

Dealing with difficult behaviours/rituals

- don't avoid, but approach difficult experiences
- remember, the best way to overcome your fear of something is to face it
- do daily relaxation – it will keep your anxiety levels down and keep your thoughts calm
- do relaxation before a difficult task
- organise your tasks and goals – give yourself plenty of time to do them
- choosing goals: – make them realistic and achievable
  – make goals and steps to them specific; what? where? when? with whom?
  – break up the goal into small steps
  – give yourself a time scale
- use recording sheets to plan and monitor your tasks
- try breathing exercises if you are in the middle of a task and it's getting the better of you
- reward yourself after achieving your task, look at the positive points even if it wasn't completed. Tell someone else about your achievement

---

Dealing with distressing thoughts

- let the thought drift through your mind when it comes out of the blue (i.e. when you're not doing a specific task)
- use distraction – switch to a pre-arranged thought pattern, e.g. imagine yourself eating your favourite meal
- use thought stopping – block the thought, say stop!, no! to yourself
- during tasks, use coping thoughts and rational answers
- coping thoughts – one step at a time
  – just think about what you have to do
  – I'll just slow down until I feel better
  – the fear will pass, I know it doesn't last long
  – I've done this before, so I can do it again
  – I know it's never as bad as I think it will be
  – I'll have a go anyway, just give it a try
  – if I stick at this, I know next time will be easier
- rational answers come from a logical assessment of the situation
  – what evidence have I got to support these thoughts?
  – these thoughts are 'old' thoughts, they belong in the past
- tell yourself that each time you manage something, that's one more piece of evidence that you *can* do it without a disaster happening

9
Self-help

This chapter is intended for use by patients, and contains ideas and hints on how to control anxiety, with details of strategies outlined in the preceding chapters, as well as helpful addresses, contacts and patient books (*see* Appendix 1). It is expected that GPs photocopy the following pages and give out relevent sections to suitable patients with anxiety problems.

Patients with mild to moderate anxiety problems, who are motivated and with sufficient understanding, should be encouraged to try out the following self-help techniques. Enabling them to develop an active, self-help approach will increase their feelings of confidence and control, and hopefully prevent exacerbation of their problem and referral to specialist mental health professionals.

All the methods described in this chapter can be used in conjunction with the cognitive-behaviour methods already described in each relevant chapter.

Ways you can help yourself

Your doctor has already discussed your particular problems with you and feels that anxiety is contributing to the way you feel and some of the difficulties in your life. There are ways you can begin to help yourself to overcome your anxiety problems. The following pages give you some suggestions of simple strategies you can learn which are known to be effective in anxiety. Many of these are taught by mental health nurses and psychologists, but it is worth you trying to learn them yourself first, before thinking about asking to see a therapist.

Learning to cope with anxiety usually requires a range of personal adjustments:

- recognition of personal causes and effects of anxiety

- reduction of anxiety in relationships, at work, and during leisure
- regular nutrition and exercise
- limitation of alcohol, tobacco and drugs
- learning relaxation skills
- learning how to control your breathing pattern
- practical management of time and activities
- the development of problem-solving strategies and social supports.

Many people discover their own ways of controlling the symptoms of anxiety without the help of doctors or other health professions. Firstly, you can learn how to reduce continuing life stresses, usually by making social or practical changes in your life. These strategies will be outlined first. Secondly, the various self-help methods of countering the symptoms of anxiety will be described.

Where available, voluntary agencies can play a very important role in helping people to help themselves. Addresses of relevant voluntary agencies, groups and self-help books are included in Appendix 1, p. 222.

General advice for patients coping with anxiety or panic includes:

- wait and the feelings will pass
- practise some of the strategies described. Use them whenever you feel panicky
- start by taking a deep breath in and then slowing down your breathing pattern
- try to distract yourself from panicky thoughts as this will stop you adding to the panic
- as the panicky feeling subsides, plan something pleasant to do next

Ten rules for coping with panic

1 Remember that the anxiety feelings are nothing more than an exaggeration of the **normal** bodily reactions to stress

2 They are not in the least harmful or dangerous – just unpleasant. Nothing worse than these feelings will happen to you

3 Stop adding to your panic with negative thoughts about what is happening and where it might lead; don't dwell on your bodily symptoms, making them seem worse than they are. Keep your thoughts in perspective. Don't catastrophise

4 Notice what is really happening around you right now, not what you fear might happen

5 The fear will reach a peak and then decrease. So, just give the fear time to pass, without fighting it, or running away from it. Just accept it and it will go away

6 Notice that once you begin to replace negative thoughts with positive, coping thoughts, the fear starts to fade away

7 Remember that the aim of approaching difficult situations is to learn how to cope with fear – without avoiding it. Each time is an opportunity to make progress

8 Think about the progress you have made so far, despite all the difficulties, and how pleased you will be when you succeed this time

9 When you begin to feel better, look around you, and start to plan what to do next

10 Then, when you are ready to go on, start off in an easy, relaxed way – there's no need for effort or hurry

Problem-solving skills

A problem-solving approach, like that described below, may be used to define exactly what stresses may be contributing to your anxiety problem and how to devise a plan to cope with it. Although some stresses cannot be fully resolved in this way, there is usually some degree of improvement in coping abilities and efforts, so that the overall impact of stress is reduced.

Put your worrying to a constructive purpose. Rather than endlessly focusing on your problems, pick out one or two that seem really important and make specific plans to resolve them. You may find it helpful to do this with a friend. Sit down with a sheet of paper and a pencil and go through the following steps, making notes as you go:

- write down exactly what the problem is

- list five or six possible solutions to the problem – write down any ideas that occur to you, not merely 'good' ideas

- weigh up the good and bad points of each idea in turn

- choose the solution that best fits your needs

- plan the steps you would take to achieve the solution

- reassess your efforts after carrying out your plan – praise all your efforts

- if you are unsuccessful, start again with a new plan.

A 'problem solving-sheet' is provided to help you with this process.

Rethinking the experience

- *List every feature of the experience.* 'I'm sweating . . . the hairs on my arm are standing on end . . . my heart is pounding hard . . . 110 per minute . . . I think I'm going to start screaming . . . my legs feel like jelly . . . I'm going to pass out.' Write these sensations down on a card.

- *Talk yourself into 'staying with' the feelings.* Tell yourself exactly how you feel, then remind yourself that the feelings will reach a peak and then subside. It is anxiety making you feel so scared; you are not in any real danger.

- *Relabel your experiences.* Imagine you are playing an energetic sport and that this accounts for your pounding heart, rapid breathing and feelings of excitement.

- *Think catastrophic thoughts.* Think of the worst possible thing that could happen to you, e.g. collapsing, screaming, etc. Plan exactly how you would cope in the slight probability of it actually happening.

Next time it will be easier to cope with the feelings, and with practice and self-monitoring you will find that you are beginning to control and overcome your tension, worry and panic.

Problem-solving sheet

Problem: _____

_____

_____

_____

List all possible solutions and note the good and bad points of each:

Solution 1 _____

Good points: _____ Bad points: _____

_____ _____

_____ _____

_____ _____

Solution 2 _____

Good points: _____ Bad points: _____

_____ _____

_____ _____

_____ _____

Solution 3 _____

Good points: _____ Bad points: _____

_____ _____

_____ _____

_____ _____

Solution 4 _____

Good points: _____ Bad points: _____

_____ _____

_____ _____

_____ _____

_____ _____

Choose the best solution and plan out the steps to achieve it:

Step 1_____

Step 2_____

Step 3_____

Step 4_____

Rushing and posture

You should plan your timetable in advance in order to avoid rushing, as feeling under pressure often leads to anxiety. You will probably find that you get just as much done by taking things gently. When taking a break, you should sit in a comfortable, relaxed posture – not hunched on the edge of a chair.

A good habit to develop is to 'scan' your body for signs of tension or anxiety at certain times throughout the day. Each person will have a particular body part that is vulnerable to tension, i.e. shoulders, neck, forehead, stomach. You can then apply your relaxation to that particular body part as soon as you feel the tension beginning.

Exercise, diet and sleep

Another priority is to ensure adequate exercise, diet and sleep. Alcohol, tobacco and non-prescribed drugs should be avoided. These are often addictive and can increase rather than relieve stress.

Exercise

Exercise is the only way to keep the body trim and fit. We all need some regular exercise, preferably daily. This might amount to no more than a pleasant 15-minute walk in the fresh air, but it could be more. At the very least, you will be more likely to feel physically and mentally relaxed, to get a refreshing sleep and have your appetite stimulated. The important thing is that the exercise chosen should be pleasurable. Whatever method of exercise is chosen, the following points need to be borne in mind:

- warm up by stretching or running on the spot for 2–3 minutes, before beginning exercising;
- build up slowly and do not overextend yourself – always exercising within the limits of comfort – let your rate of breathing be the guide;
- if you feel excessively tired stop and rest – there is always tomorrow;
- when stopping exercise cool down gradually and slowly to avoid stiffness;

- exercise sessions three times a week for about 20 minutes at a pace that keeps you moderately puffed, not gasping for breath, are the best for stimulating the muscles and circulation.

Diet

The main principles are to eat less fat and fatty foods, especially those containing saturated fats and cholesterol. Increase dietary fibre by eating more whole-grain cereals, pulses, and fresh fruit and vegetables, cut down on sugar and salt. Change a few products at a time and add new foods rather than just cutting out those that are 'prohibited'. Changing diet should not be torture, it should be fun. Too much tea or coffee can be overstimulating and excessive alcohol is no friend to good health.

Sleep

If you have difficulties sleeping, you should make a daily diary or record of your sleep pattern. This will allow you to see whether the problem is as bad as you think and whether it is getting worse, better or staying the same. It will also help you to judge whether anything you have tried in order to improve sleep has had the desired effect. Start by recording the times you are asleep in each 24–hour period, and the quality of each sleep, for example is it restful, fitful or dozing? Make a note of whether the sleep is in bed, in a chair or in front of the television. Finally, note whether you tried anything to help sleep, for example, a hot drink, relaxation or a prescribed drug. Catnaps in an armchair in front of the television and on the train can make up for sleep lost during the night.

Stress reduction

Stress in our lives adds to our worries. The first step in getting rid of excess stress is to be aware of what is causing us stress.

Next, there are some basic changes you can make in your life to protect you from many everyday stresses. Decide on one or two of these changes each week. Don't try to change everything at once! Take it gradually, that's the best way to make lasting changes. Remember that breaking bad habits takes time and perseverence.

Advice on getting to sleep

- Try not to worry about the amount of sleep you are missing. This only makes things worse
- Go to bed at a regular time
- If you go to bed too early you should go to bed a quarter of an hour later each evening for a week or so until sleep improves
- If you wake tired in the morning try bringing bedtime forward a quarter of an hour each night until you wake refreshed and not too early
- Avoid sleeping during the day so that you are more tired at bedtime
- Try eating the evening meal at a regular time several hours before going to bed
- Take some regular exercise. A quiet stroll in the evening will help relaxation and make you feel more tired
- Avoid stimulating exercise before bedtime
- Avoid stimulating drinks and tobacco close to bedtime
- Reduce intake of tea, coffee or cola to no more than two to three drinks daily and have the last drink several hours before bedtime
- A warm bath may also help relaxation before bed
- A regular routine at bedtime helps you get into the frame of mind for sleep
- Do not listen to the radio or read in bed unless these are particularly useful ways of helping you relax
- Avoid sedative drugs and alcohol at bedtime
- Try the relaxation technique described later while lying comfortably in bed
- If unable to sleep because of worrying: try getting up, taking a piece of paper and pen, writing down exactly what the problem is, making a list of every possible solution to the problem, choosing a solution that you can begin next day and planning exactly how you would carry out the plan
- Do not lie awake for longer than 30 minutes. Get up and find a constructive activity

Strategies for coping with stress – identifying the source of your stress:

- This may be obvious to you, e.g. colleagues, money worries, work, relationships – if not obvious, think about difficult aspects of your life
  - **Try to be honest with yourself**
- Your stress may be due to conflict: not wanting to do something you feel you ought to do; wanting to do incompatible things; feeling ambivalent towards someone
  - **Try to sort out your feelings**
- Your stress may be due to feeling helpless in a particular situation
  - **Try to assess realistically whether there is anything you can do**
- Your stress may be due to a situation that makes you feel bad about yourself (inadequate, bored, guilty, etc.)
  - **Try to change the way you see the situation**
- Your stress may be due to feeling pressurised, perhaps because you feel you have to prove yourself or think there is no one else to carry the load
  - **Either way, try to share or shed some of the responsibility**
- Your stress may be due to trying to be someone or something that is not really you
  - **Ask yourself why?**
- Your stress may be due merely to fears of what might happen or even vague fears you have never put into words
  - **As yourself: fact or fiction?**
- Your stress may be due to a combination of factors, some related, some not
  - **Try to separate them out and see how they interact**

Basic stress-avoidance rules

General

- Learn to relax: use your relaxation tape. Make sure you put relaxation into practice in your everyday life

- Eat properly: avoid too much fat and sugar. Eat sensibly. Introduce more fresh fruit, vegetables and fibre. Eat to enjoy your food, but don't over-eat

- Smoke and drink in moderation. Try to cut down on drinking and stop smoking (see section on stopping smoking)

- Identify sources of stress and deal with them one at a time. Don't rush in trying to settle all your problems at once. Make a list and patiently work through them

- Get up a few minutes earlier in the morning, allowing yourself to wake up and prepare for the day. Use this time to take the 'rush' and 'bustle' out of life

- Don't try to do everything and be everything to everybody. Get your priorities right – make sure you do the vital things first and leave the inessential for later

- Listen to others. Don't try to do all the talking, narrow the conversation to what interests you most

- Learn to say 'no'. Don't simply take on everything that people expect of you. Examine your committments over the last week – how many could have been passed on?

- Set appropriate schedules for your family, work, personal interests and social life. Allocate time and opportunities to each area. All areas of your life are important, don't just work and then cram in everything else into whatever time is left over. Plan specifics each week

- Set realistic life goals and ambitions: don't simply do what you do because 'it's always been done that way'. Decide what it is you want from life and realistically plan for this

- Don't set out to win everything. Don't beat others at traffic lights, don't overtake unnecessarily. Make sure you do your best where it really matters, but don't push yourself in other circumstances

- Don't take 'I have to' for granted. Look at all your responsibilities and duties and see if you really have to do all these things

Work

- Don't be at the mercy of your environment. Cut out those inessential phone calls and interruptions. Concentrate on the things that must be done. Don't be available to people at all times
- Learn to delegate
- Pace your work during the day by taking short rest periods. Don't work through the whole of the day, take 10 minutes morning and afternoon for total relaxation
- Set yourself appropriate schedules. Don't rush around frantically. Pace yourself, go at a steady rate. If you can't do everything without rushing, then you're doing too much!
- Be tidy and orderly. Untidiness tends to create a sense of time urgency and important things get missed
- Take clear lunch breaks. Don't snatch a sandwich while working. Sit down, eat in a relaxed way, enjoying your lunch. Take a good half hour for this. If possible, go away from your work to eat. Take a walk or sit in the sunshine
- Don't procrastinate: plan things in advance, don't leave it to the last minute

Leisure

- Physical fitness: do a little light exercise 2–3 times per week. Don't push yourself too hard, simply try to avoid being too sedentary
- Programme leisure time. Don't just 'flop' when you finish work. Take up specific activities and exercise. Exercise actually helps with tension, relaxation and sleep problems. It also gives you a sense of well-being and more energy
- Programme some time for yourself each week, it needn't be long, but make sure its not forgotten. Spend the time thinking, taking stock of your life and whatever you enjoy
- Don't see traditions and ceremonies as time wasting. 'Take time to smell the flowers', appreciate the good things in your life, be thankful. Go and look at a church building, lean on a fence and admire the view, etc. This helps put your life into perspective.

Breaking bad habits

Smoking tobacco, drinking excess alcohol and taking drugs of dependence (sometimes even those prescribed by the doctor, if not carefully monitored) are habits that will not help you tackle your anxiety problem. They are 'false friends' as they give the illusion of temporary relief from stress, while in reality making it more difficult for you to directly address your problems.

People under stress sometimes attempt to cope, either deliberately or unconsciously, by using these substances to deal with their symptoms or to withstand the pressure they feel.

Alcohol

Alcohol in moderation may be a pleasure, but it is a potentially addictive drug with many subtle and complicated effects. Any long-standing stressful situation invites the serious risk of heavy drinking and eventual dependence on alcohol, which can ruin marriages, family and social life, careers and health.

The main signs that you may be developing a dependence on alcohol are listed below. Not all these signs may be present and they may occur to variable degrees in different people:

- awareness of a compulsion to drink

- developing a daily drinking pattern

- drinking takes priority over other activities

- tolerance for alcohol changes – usually increases at first but eventually falls

- repeated symptoms of alcohol withdrawal – nausea, headache, nervousness, shaking, sweating, tenseness, jitteriness, being 'on-edge'

- relief or avoidance of withdrawal symptoms by further drinking

- rapid return of the features of dependence after a period of abstinence.

Safe levels of drinking are difficult to define precisely for each person, and depend on factors such as gender, body size and constitution. Current advice is that the sensible limit for men should be no more than

21 units a week and, for women, up to 14 units a week. In both cases, the units should be spread throughout the week, with two or three drink-free days. The equivalents to a unit of alcohol are listed below:

- half a pint of beer, cider or lager (of normal strength)
- a single measure of spirits
- a small glass of wine.

How much is too much?

For men, 36 units and for women 22 units or more in 1 week. It is worth remembering that, on average, it takes 1 hour for the body to get rid of each unit of alcohol. A man who drinks four or more pints a day (56 units a week), or a woman who drinks more than five small glasses of wine a day (35 units a week) is at great risk of developing an alcohol-related problem.

Using the guidelines opposite, you may find it helpful to involve a supportive relative or friend to join you in reducing your drinking.

Smoking

The most common reason cigarette smokers give for not stopping smoking is that it helps them cope with stress. Nicotine provides short-term relief from feelings of stress, but smoking is not a good long-term strategy for dealing with stress. This is because, once the nicotine effect wears off, there is a 'rebound' effect, whereby stress levels increase even more. Smoking will not solve the problems that make you tense; smoking brings its own anxieties. Quite apart from the serious health risks associated with smoking, smokers can experience the following anxieties: worries about what others think of them, lowered self-esteem, worries about enforced abstinence (e.g. aeroplane flights), cravings for the next cigarette, worries about the effects on their children, higher insurance and mortgage premiums . . .

The most important step to giving up smoking is the decision that you really do want to stop.

Once you make that decision for yourself, you're halfway there. If you feel you need some help, consider some form of nicotine-replacement therapy: from nicotine gum to patches. This works by allowing the body

Tips to help cut down drinking

- Reduce the overall amount by stopping drinking at certain times, e.g. lunch time, and do something else instead
- Allow yourself only one alcoholic drink an hour at any drinking session
- Avoid drinking in 'rounds' if this means you will drink more than you wish
- Have a long soft drink to quench your thirst before starting on alcohol
- Remember that what others drink is irrelevant to your own health
- Try to find some non-alcoholic alternative in drinking situations
- Add mixers to wines and spirits to increase the volume and help slow down consumption
- Keep yourself busy, plan activities that will keep your mind off drink
- Avoid reminders of drinking and, whenever possible, places where alcohol will be consumed or people will offer you a drink. Plan avoidance action for times when you are confronted by these particular situations
- Keep a record of how well you are doing in reducing drinking. Don't think you've failed if you slip back for a day; take a longer term view of your success. Reward yourself for your success and persistance with something you enjoy apart from alcohol

to adjust gradually to lower amounts of nicotine. Remember though, nicotine replacements are aids to you giving up and not cures.

Remember that you had no need to smoke before you became hooked. The first cigarette always tastes awful, and smokers have to be dedicated to become addicted in the first place. The most annoying part is that non-smokers do not seem to be missing out; smokers keep smoking to achieve the same state of tranquility as non-smokers, so you can learn to find other ways of achieving this too.

As well as the 'sensible' reasons for stopping, ask yourself:

- what is smoking doing for me?
- do I actually enjoy it?
- are there other ways of achieving the relaxing effects of smoking?

Six steps to giving up smoking

1 Decide that you really want to do it, and realise that you can achieve your goal. Others have done it before you and you have as much will-power as anyone else. It is only indecision that makes giving up more difficult

2 Recognise the fact that you have been addicted to nicotine, but that withdrawal is not as painful as you think. It only takes about 3 weeks to rid the body of 99% of the nicotine

3 Look forward to the freedom that awaits you. Do not be afraid of losing the prop you have been brainwashed into believeing you cannot do without. Smoking enslaves you, preventing you from achieving the peace and confidence you used to have

4 Pick a day to stop smoking completely. Remember, there is no such thing as 'just one'. Smoking is a drug addiction and a chain reaction. By moping about the one cigarette, you will be punishing yourself needlessly

5 Watch out for smokers – they may feel threatened by the fact that you have given up, and may try to tempt you back. Try giving up with a friend, going to places where you won't be reminded of smoking. Find other interests and activities to distract you and keep your hands occupied

6 No longer see yourself as a smoker, you've changed your identity. Take pride in joining the growing legions of non-smokers! Keep reminding yourself that you're not giving up something, but gaining. Keep focused on the enormous, positive gains to be had by not smoking

It is often the fear of giving up smoking that prevents people from making that vital decision. The effects of withdrawal are not difficult to handle. There is no physical pain, merely an empty, restless feeling, the sense of something missing. If withdrawal is prolonged, the smoker can become nervous, insecure, lacking in confidence and irritable. This is the worst you may feel, and if you stick with it past this stage, the rest gets a lot easier. Many people get to this stage and go back to smoking, so the next time they 'try' to give up, they remember the bad times. Try to remember that 'the darkest hour is just before dawn', so success is just around the corner!

There is a national telephone helpline to give you the encouagement and support you may need in giving up: Smokers' QUITLINE (Free-phone) 0800 002200, open 9–11 a.m., daily. They provide telephone counselling, send out free information packs and can refer you to local Stop Smoking groups.

Anxiety management techniques

The main techniques for controlling anxiety are **relaxation, breathing retraining, distraction** and **answering your anxious thoughts**. Many of you may well have attempted to use these before coming to your doctor; indeed, these techniques are often seen as things recommended by 'common sense'. However, they are not always easy to apply and need to be practised regularly and tried out in a range of situations if they are to become really useful in your everyday life. All the techniques are harder to use at high levels of anxiety, and so should be first learnt when you are relaxed and able to concentrate.

Appropriate self-monitoring sheets, diaries, etc. are included for your use in Appendix 2. Your doctor will be able to guide you to the most suitable techniques and advise you if you have problems understanding what to do.

Relaxation training

One of the simplest ways of achieving relaxation is through planning enjoyable and relaxing activities and planning regular breaks in busy schedules. Most people with anxiety will also benefit from more formal training in relaxation techniques. Progressive muscular relaxation is the method recommended here.

Relaxation training for patients

Relaxation is a useful technique to practice when you feel tense or worried. Read the instructions and familiarise yourself with them before having a go. Be patient and give yourself several attempts before expecting the full benefits. It can take time to learn how to relax. Keep a diary of your efforts, so that you can follow your progress. A friend or relative may help you to stick to the task, particularly when progress seems slow and difficult.

Preparation. Sit in a comfortable chair or lie down somewhere comfortable in a quiet, warm room where you will not be interrupted. If you are sitting, take off your shoes, uncross your legs, and rest your arms on the arms of the chair. If you are lying down, lie on your back with your arms at your sides. If necessary use a comfortable pillow for your head. Close your eyes and be aware of your body. Notice how you are breathing and where the muscular tensions are. Make sure you are comfortable.

Breathing. Start to breathe slowly and deeply, expanding your abdomen as you breathe in, then raising your rib cage to let more air in, until your lungs are filled right to the top. Hold your breath for a couple of seconds and then breathe out slowly, allowing your rib cage and stomach to relax, and empty your lungs completely. **Do not strain**, with practice it will become much easier. Keep this slow, deep, rhythmic breathing going throughout your relaxation session.

Relaxing. After about 5 minutes, when you have your breathing pattern established, start the following sequence, tensing each part of the body on an in-breath, holding your breath for 6 seconds while you keep your muscles tense, then relax and breathe out at the same time. The muscle groups should be tensed for a few seconds, then totally relaxed.

    i   Curl your toes hard and press your feet down.
    ii   Press your heels down and bend your feet up.
   iii   Tense your calf muscles.
   iv   Tense your thigh muscles, straightening your knees and making your legs stiff.
    v   Make your buttocks tight.
   vi   Tense your stomach as if to receive a punch.
  vii   Bend your elbows and tense the muscles of your arms.
 viii   Hunch your shoulders and press your head back into the cushion or pillow.

ix Clench your jaws, frown and screw up your eyes really tight.
x Tense all your muscles together.

Remember to breathe deeply, and be aware when you relax of the feeling of physical well-being and heaviness spreading through your body.

Pleasant imagery. After you have gone through the whole sequence **(i–x)** and you are still breathing slowly and deeply, try to imagine yourself in a favourite place. This might be lying on a deserted beach with palm trees around you, in a beautiful spring meadow with birds singing in the trees, in a lovely garden surrounded by beautiful flowers, or in a rocking chair next to a warm winter fire. The place you choose should be pleasant and peaceful, a special place for you. Put effort into using all your senses to feel as if you are really there, seeing things in your mind's eye as clearly as possible. Concentrate on the sounds you would hear, the warm feeling on your skin, the smells around you. Do not hold your breathing during this time, continue to breathe as you have been doing. See yourself in your special place, relaxed and content with yourself.

Lastly, tell yourself that when you open your eyes you will be perfectly relaxed but alert.

Short routine

When you have become familiar with this technique, if you want to relax at any time when you have only a few minutes, do the sequence in a shortened form, leaving out some muscle groups, but always working from your feet upwards. For example, you might do numbers **i**, **vi**, **viii** and **x** if you do not have time to do the whole sequence.

You may find it easier to make a relaxation tape for yourself. Ask a friend or relative to help by reading the instructions above into a tape recorder. Alternatively, there are now a wide choice of relaxation tapes available in the shops. If you would like to try these, we recommend that you check the tape is using the **progressive muscular relaxation** technique, as this is the most effective. However, gentle music, seascape sounds or birdsong tapes can also be peaceful and help you to imagine you are in a pleasant place whilst you are relaxing.

Relaxation is one of the best ways you can learn to control your anxiety. You should practise applying relaxation in different settings so that you can use it when in a stressful situation. This means practising relaxation while sitting, standing and carrying on with everyday activities as these are situations in which you will need to control your anxiety. With time, you will learn to notice your own early signs of anxiety, and use these as cues to relax.

Quick release of tension

Whenever you feel anxious, panicky or uptight . . .

1 Let your breath out (don't breathe in first)
2 Take in a slow, gentle breath; hold it for a second
3 Let it go with a loud sigh of relief
4 Drop your shoulders at the same time and relax your hands
5 Make sure your teeth are not clenched together
6 If you have to speak, speak more slowly and in a lower tone of voice

---

Controlling breathing

Breathing retraining

Rapid anxious breathing makes you tremble, feel dizzy and light-headed, produces a thumping heart and a tingling sensation in the hands and feet. Panic attacks often begin by people having difficulty breathing, which leads to these bodily symptoms which in turn make you feel anxious. These symptoms can be quickly controlled by slow, shallow breathing at the rate of 8–12 breaths per minute.

The 6-second breath

Controlling the rate of breathing is one of the most important things you can do to stop anxiety from getting out of control. You should practise breathing one breath every 6 seconds, breathing in through the nose for 3 seconds and out of the mouth for the next 3 seconds. This can be in stages, e.g. in–in–in, out–out–out and so forth.

This '6-second breath' can be extended to 8 or 10 seconds, and can be used anywhere and any time when you start to feel anxious. It is useful to practise this technique a few times per day when you are calm so that it is well rehearsed for a time when it is needed.

Another useful breathing technique is to breathe into a paper bag. Exactly why this works is a little complicated, but basically, breathing in your used air increases the levels of carbon dioxide. This works to slow down your rate of breathing and reduce some of your anxiety symptoms.

Making sure you are breathing from your abdomen rather than your chest is another way to ensure that you are breathing properly. You can practise this using the instructions below.

Rhythmical abdominal breathing

1 Sit or lie down in a comfortable position with your back straight. Bend your knees and have your feet about 8 inches apart. Close your eyes. Let your body be relaxed without tension, your face smooth and relaxed, shoulders loose and chest floppy

2 Put the palms of your hands on your abdomen (tummy area) so that the tips of the middle fingers of both hands touch over your navel

3 Now breathe in through the nose, slowly and evenly, filling the lungs. Notice that as you breathe in your ribcage expands and at the same time your abdomen rises, lifting your hands so that your fingertips separate slightly

4 Now breathe out, slowly and evenly, emptying the lungs fully. Notice that as you breathe out your abdomen falls so that your fingertips touch again, and your ribcage moves in

5 As you breathe in you can start counting to three, then as you breathe out also count to three. This way your in-breath and your out-breath are the same length, and your breathing becomes an even rhythm. As you practise this you can increase your counting to 4 . . . 5 . . . and then 6, when you breathe in and out

---

Distraction

Paying attention to anxiety symptoms in your body keeps the vicious circle going, causing you to worry about what is happening, which makes the symptoms worse and worse. Distraction reverses this process, and is useful as a short-term strategy for controlling anxiety. However, it is unhelpful in the long-term if used as a way of avoiding symptoms or reducing exposure.

To help when you are feeling anxious, you can learn to make yourself

The relaxing sigh

During the day you probably catch yourself sighing or yawning. This is a sign that you are not getting enough oxygen; sighing and yawning are your body's way of remedying this. A sigh releases a bit of tension and can be practised at will as a means of relaxing.

1 Sit or stand up straight

2 Sigh deeply, letting out a sound of deep relief as the air rushes out of your lungs

3 Don't think about inhaling – just let the air come in naturally

4 Repeat this process 8–12 times whenever you feel the need for it and experience the sensation of relaxation

concentrate on what is happening around you, rather than your anxiety or what is happening in your body. You should choose something that engages your full attention. Mental activity such as a crossword puzzle is acceptable to some; physical activity and keeping occupied is more helpful to others. Try some of the following ways to turn your attention from anxious symptoms and thoughts.

1 **Concentrating** on what is going on around you (e.g. by counting the branches on a tree, cars in the street or things beginning with a certain letter). Choose something that engages your full attention. There are many possible variations on this theme.

2 **Mental activity** such as remembering a list, reciting a poem or doing mental arithmetic (e.g. counting backwards from 100 in threes).

3 **Physical activity** such as walking, gardening or ironing. Keeping yourself occupied helps distract you from your thoughts.

Controlling upsetting thoughts

Upsetting thoughts only make you feel more anxious. The first step is to find out exactly what the upsetting thoughts are. This is difficult because upsetting thoughts are automatic and come and go so quickly. Therefore, you need to learn how to recognise and identify them. You should try to write them down exactly as they occur when you are feeling anxious. Once you can 'tune in' to what thoughts are going through your head, you can then examine the thoughts carefully and identify those that are exaggerated or unrealistic. (For example, 'I didn't get the job so nobody will employ me', 'I feel tense about talking at the meeting and I will make a hash of it' or 'I shouted at the kids so I am a lousy mum'.)

There are positive and more reasonable alternatives to all these thoughts. Try to write them down and then look at some of your own thoughts and try to find more reasonable alternatives. This is difficult at first but with practice, and a bit of help, it becomes easier. Anxious thoughts can come before a situation, when you feel the anxiety symptoms or after the situation. There are some questions below to help you examine your anxious thoughts and come up with rational answers. Obviously, not all questions will work for every thought; you have to try them out to see which ones work for you most often.

Questions to help you examine your anxious thoughts

- What evidence do I have for this thought? Is there another way of looking at things?

- How would someone else think about my situation? How would I think about someone else in this situation?

- Are my judgements based on how I felt rather than what I did? e.g. feeling anxious, but actually coped well with it.

- Am I setting myself an unrealistic or unotainable standard? Am I trying to be perfect or deal with everything well?

- Am I forgetting relevant facts or overemphasising irrelevant facts? i.e. do I forget previous successes and focus on infrequent failures?

- Am I thinking in 'all or nothing' terms? Come to a compromise, settle for grey areas rather than black or white extremes.

- So what if it does happen? What would be so bad about that? Let yourself consider the worst; it will probably be less disastrous and less likely than you assume.

- Am I underestimating what I can do to deal with the situation? How have I dealt with hard situations in the past? What skills and resources do I have to tackle this present challenge?

- Am I overestimating the likelihood of danger in this situation? Am I letting my anxiety stop me thinking rationally?

Some thought-recording sheets are included in Appendix 2 to help you to identify and modify your thoughts throughout treatment. If you have difficulty understanding what to do, your doctor will help you.

Coping self-statements

You should make a list of encouraging things to say to yourself when entering a stressful situation as this will stop the pattern of anxious thoughts beginning and also make it more likely that you will cope well. Think of things you would say to your best friend in a similar situation and say them to yourself. Often we are more critical of ourselves than others, whereas we should treat ourselves with as much concern and respect as we do others.

Here are some ideas of coping self-statements, but obviously they will be more effective if you think up your own.

- 'This is just anxiety, I've gone through this before. All I need to do is stay with it and it will eventually go away.'

- 'Take one step at a time; what is the first thing I have to do – start breathing properly. In 1 . . . 2 . . . 3 . . ., out 1 . . . 2 . . . 3.'

- 'Don't focus on the symptoms or your fear, it helps to distract yourself – how many red things can I see?'

- 'I can cope with this. I have learnt things I can do to keep my anxiety levels down. They have worked before and will work again for me now.'

Thinking in this way will make you feel stronger and more able to cope with whatever situation you are facing. Direct yourself to coping strategies you have learnt and practised. Keep yourself from thinking the worst. This will increase your confidence and make you feel more in control of things – that there is something practical you can do to help yourself, rather than letting yourself feel weak and helpless.

Dealing with avoidance and loss of confidence

Avoiding places or certain situations because they make you anxious seems at first to make sense. But in fact, it makes things harder for you, because each time you avoid doing something, it makes it more likely you will avoid it the next time. The more things you avoid, the narrower your life becomes, until you may eventually feel like a prisoner in your own home. However, this problem can be overcome by gradually getting back into the habit of doing things which build up your confidence.

Once you realise that avoiding things actually keeps your anxiety going, you are ready to face up to some of the things that make you anxious. You can then learn that in fact, you are able to cope, as long as you use skills such as breathing, relaxation, distraction and controlling your thoughts.

Work your way through the steps given in the box below to plan how to face up to things you avoid, or situations that make you feel anxious.

Steps for facing difficult situations

1 Make a list of the situations that are avoided or lead to anxiety

2 Arrange these in order according to how difficult it would be to face each one

3 Select the easiest item on the list as the first target to practise. Describe the target you are aiming for very clearly in writing

4 Make a plan of things you can do to keep your anxiety down, such as distraction, breathing and relaxation. You may want to write some 'coping thoughts' on a card to take with you

5 See how well you can cope with the easiest item on your list. Remember, your anxiety is bound to go up, but if you stay in the situation, it will come down again. Repeat this item many times until it can be done without difficulty

6 Move on to the next item on the list and so on

This is a simplified version of what therapists call a graded hierarchy, or 'fear ladder'. A sheet to help you plan this exercise is included in Appendix 2. Again, if you have difficulty with this, your GP will be able to advise you.

To be helpful, practice must be regular, frequent and for fairly long periods. If something appears too difficult, break it down into smaller steps or for a shorter time and gradually build up the practice time.

Do not be put off if you feel a bit worse to begin with – this is almost inevitable. Be prepared to put some effort into regaining your confidence. It is common to think you are not making any progress at

Suggestions for family and friends

- Encourage the person with anxiety to **eat properly** and **to take some daily exercise**, such as walking

- Give **reminders to practise their relaxation exercises daily**. This is especially important after a stressful day, so that tension does not build up

- When they become anxious, help them by encouraging them to use their **relaxation, breathing** and **self-talk skills.** Reassure them that the **anxiety is temporary and will pass**

- It is not helpful to suggest that they 'pull themselves together' – **they would if they could.** Statements like these undermine confidence. Instead, it is better to tell them you feel they are up to the task, encouraging them to try

- Try to concentrate on the positive side of things – talk together about the ways in which they have coped with anxiety. **Remind them of their successes**, however small they may seem, rather than the 'failures'

- Try very hard **not to give in** if they want you to check things, do things for them or help them avoid some activity. Help them regain their independence by being **gentle yet firm**

- Try not to be overcritical, people with anxiety are **sensitive** and **easily hurt**. Rather help them by encouraging them, telling them they can do it, etc.

- You can **become involved with them in the various self-help activities** and ideas outlined in these pages. Make sure you offer your help, but allow them to decide what they want to try. With your **gentle enthusiasm and encouragement** they will find it easier to make a start

- Remember to **allow plenty of time for jobs** such as shopping, outings, etc. Plan ahead so that jobs are spread out evenly over a few days. A hectic schedule will only build up high levels of anxiety and tension

- People who express ideas about **not wanting to live** should be taken seriously and a doctor or other professional helper should be involved

- Try not to take to heart what the person says if it seems hurtful – usually it is **unintentional**

first, and to underrate your achievements. Therefore, it is helpful to have a member of the family or a trusted friend give you encouragement and help you plan your targets.

If your problems are to do with checking or irrational thoughts, there are some relevent sheets and helpful tips in Appendix 2 which your GP will go over with you.

Role of family and friends

Although family and friends are often able to understand the distress caused by anxiety, it can be difficult for them to deal with it first hand, particularly if anxiety seems unreasonable, is disruptive to everyday life or becomes prolonged.

Every anxious person and every situation are different but the following suggestions may be helpful to the family and friends of someone who is anxious.

References

American Psychiatric Association (1994) *Diagnostic and Statistical Manual of Mental Disorders* (4e). American Psychiatric Association Press, Washington, DC.

Bebbington PE (1998) Epidemiology of obsessive-compulsive disorder. *British Journal of Psychiatry*. **173** (Suppl 35): 2–6.

Blake D (1990) A clinician rating scale for assessing current and lifetime PTSD: the CAPS-I. *Behav Therapist*. **18**, 187–8.

Balestrieri M, Williams P and Wilkinson G (1988) Specialist mental health treatment in general practice: a meta-analysis. *Psychological Medicine*. **18**: 711–17.

Beaumont G (1991) Anxiolytics in practice: minimizing the problems. *Prescriber*. **28**: 43–7.

Braun P, Greenberg D, Dasberg H and Lerer B (1990) Core symptoms of PTSD unimproved by alprazolam treatment. *Journal of Clinical Psychiatry*. **51**: 236–8.

Carnwath T and Miller D (1986*) Behavioural Psychotherapy in Primary Care: a practice manual*. Harcourt Brace Jovanovich, London.

Clark D (1986) A cognitive approach to panic. *Behav Res Therapy*. **24**: 461–70.

Cooper B (1965) A study of 100 chronic psychiatric patients identified in general practice. *The British Journal of Psychiatry*. **3**: 595–605.

Cox T (1988) *Stress*. Macmillan Education, London.

Creamer M, Burgess P and Pattison P (1992) Reaction to trauma: a cognitive processing model. *J Abnorm Psychol*. **101**: 453–9.

Davidson J, Smith R and Kudler H (1989) Validity and reliability of the DSM-III criteria for post-traumatic stress disorder: experience with a structured interview. *J Ment Nerv Dis*. **177**(6): 336–41.

den Boer JA (1999) Literature review presented at European Neuro-science Conference, Madrid, March 18–20, 1999.

France R and Robson M (1986). *Behaviour Therapy in Primary Care: a practical guide*. Croon Helm, London.

Freud S (1964) Moses and monotheism. In: J Strachey (ed. and trans.) *The Standard Edition of the Complete Psychological Works of Sigmund Freud*

(Vol. 23). Hogarth Press, London. (Original work published 1937–1939.)

Gask L, McGrath G, Goldberg D and Millar T (1987) Improving the psychiatric skills of established general practitioners: evaluation of group teaching. *Med Education.* **21**: 362–68.

Gask L, Goldberg D, Lesser AL and Millar T (1988) Improving the psychiatric skills of the general practice trainee: an evaluation of a group training course. *Med Education.* **22**: 132–8.

Goldberg D and Huxley P (1980) *Mental Illness in the Community: the pathway to psychiatric care.* Tavistock Publications Ltd, London.

Goldberg D, Bridges K, Duncan Jones P and Grayson D (1988) Detecting anxiety and depression in general medical settings. *BMJ.* **297**: 897–9.

Goldberg D, Gask L and O'Dowd T (1989) The treatment of somatization: teaching techniques of reattribution. *Journal of Psychosomatic Research.* **33**: 689–95.

Greenberger D and Padesky CA (1995) *Mind Over Mood: change the way you feel by changing the way you think.* The Guilford Press, New York.

Hammarberg M (1992) PENN Inventory for post-traumatic stress disorder: psychometric properties. *Psychol Assess.* **4**(1): 67–76.

Hawton K, Salkovskis P, Kirk J and Clark D (1992) *Cognitive Behaviour Therapy for Psychiatric Problems.* Oxford University Press, Oxford.

Horowitz M (1986) *Stress Response Syndromes.* Aronson, New York.

Horowitz M, Wilner N and Alvarez W (1979) Impact of Event Scale: a measure of subjective stress. *Psychosom Med.* **41**(3): 209–18.

ICD-10 (1992) *International Classification of Diseases* (10e). World Health Organisation, Geneva.

Jenkins R, Smeeton N and Shepherd M (1988) *Classification of mental disorder in primary care.* Psychological Medicine Monograph Supplement 132. Cambridge University Press, Cambridge.

Jezzard RG (1995) Child and adolescent psychiatric disorders in general practice. *Adv Psychiat Treatment.* **1**: 184–91.

Jones JC and Barlow DH (1992) A new model of posttraumatic stress disorder: implications for the future. In: PA Saigh (ed.) *Posttraumatic stress disorder.* Macmillan, New York.

Kardiner A (1941) The traumatic neurosis of war. *Psychological Medicine Monograph (1–11).* National Research Council, Washington, DC.

Keane TM, Zimering RT and Caddell JM (1985) A behavioural formulation of posttraumatic stress disorders in Vietnam veterans. *Behav Therapist.* **8**: 9–12.

Kilpatrick DG, Veronen LJ and Resick PA (1982) Psychological sequelae to rape. In: DM Doleys, RL Meredith and AR Ciminero (eds)

Behavioural Medicine: assessment and treatment strategies. Plenum Press, New York.

Kilpatrick DG and Resnick HS (1993) Post-traumatic stress disorder associated with exposure to criminal victimization in a clinical and a community population. In: J Davidson and EB Foa (eds) *Post-traumatic Stress Disorder DSM IV and Beyond*. American Psychiatric Association, Washington DC.

Kulka RA, Schlenger WE, Fairbank RL *et al.* (1990) *Trauma and the Vietnam War generation: report of findings from the National Vietnam Veterans Readjustment Study*. Brunner Mazel, New York.

Macculloch MJ and Feldman P (1996) Eye movement desensitisation treatment utilises the positive visceral element of the investigatory reflex to inhibit the memories of post-traumatic stress disorder: a theoretical analysis. *British Journal of Psychiatry*. **169**: 571–9.

McGlone G (1998) Stress and the GP. *Psychiat Gen Pract*. Winter: 17–19.

McIvor R (1998) Post-traumatic stress disorder: the role of drug therapy. *Progress in Neurology and Psychiatry*. **2**(5): 18–21.

Mann AH, Jenkins R and Belsey E (1981) The twelve month outcome of neurotic patients in general pratice. *Psychol Med*. **11**: 535–50.

Markus AC, Murray Parkes C, Tomson P and Johnston M (1989) *Psychological Problems in General Practice*. Oxford University Press, Oxford.

Meichenbaum DH (1985) *Stress Inoculation Training*. Pergamon Press, New York.

Rachman SJ and Hodgson R (1980) *Obsessions and Compulsions*. Prentice Hall, Englewood Cliffs, NJ.

Rachman SJ (1993) Obsessions, responsibility and guilt. *Behav Res Therapy*. **31**: 149-54.

Rachman S and de Silva P (1996) *Panic Disorder: the facts*. Oxford University Press, Oxford.

Raynes NV (1979) Factors affecting the prescribing of psychotic drugs in general practice consultations. *Psychol Med*. **9**(4): 671–9.

Resick PA and Schnicke MK (1992) Cognitive processing therapy for sexual abuse victims. *J Counselling Clin Psychol*. **60**: 748–56.

Riggs DS and Foa EB (1993) Obsessive compulsive disorder. In: DH Barlow (ed) *Clinical Handbook of Psychological Disorders* (2e). The Guilford Press, New York.

Salkovskis PM (1985) Obsessional-compulsive problems: a cognitive-behavioural analysis. *Behav Res Therapy*. **23**: 571–83.

Salkovskis PM (1988) Intrusive thoughts and obsessional disorders. In: D Glasgow and N Eisenberg (eds) *Current Issues in Clinical Psychology* (Vol. 4). Gower, London.

Salkovskis PM and Warwick HMC (1988) Cognitive therapy of obsessive-compulsive disorder. In: C Perris, IM Blackburn and H Perris (eds) *The Theory and Practice of Cognitive Therapy*. Springer-Verlag, Heidelberg.

Saxena S, Brody AL, Schwartz JM and Baxter LR (1998) Neuroimaging and frontal-subcortical circuitry in obsessive-compulsive disorder. *British Journal of Psychiatry*. **173** (Suppl 35): 26–37.

Scott MJ and Stradling SG (1995) *Counselling for Post-Traumatic Stress Disorder*. Sage Publications, London.

Shapiro F (1989) Eye movement desensitisation: a new treatment for post traumatic stress disorder. *J Behaviour Ther Exp Psychiatry*. **20**: 211–17.

Shepherd M and Wilkinson G (1988) Primary care as the middle ground for psychiatric epidemiology. *Psychol Med*. **18**: 263–7.

Sibbald B, Addington-Hall J and Brenneman D (1993) Counsellors in English and Welsh general practices: their nature and distribution. *BMJ*. **306**: 29–33.

Stein G (1988) Anxiety disorders. In: G Stein and G Wilkinson (eds) *General Adult Psychiatry (Vol 1)*. Royal College of Psychiatrists/Gaskell, London.

Titchener JL (1985) Post-traumatic decline: a consequence of unresolved destructive drives. In: CR Figley (ed.) *Trauma and Its Wake: Traumatic Stress Theory Research and Intervention (Vol 2)*. Brunner Mazel, New York.

True WR, Rice J, Eisen SA *et al.* (1993) A twin study of genetic and environmental contributions to liability for post-traumatic stress symptoms. *Archives of General Psychiatry*. **50**: 257–64.

Watson CG, Juba MP, Manifold V, Kucala T and Anderson PE (1991) The PTSD interview: rationale, description, reliability, and concurrent validity or a DSM-III-based technique. *J Clin Psychol*. **47**(2): 179–88.

Wilkinson G (1988) I don't want to see a psychiatrist. *BMJ*. **297**: 1144–5.

Wilkinson G, Moore B and Moore P (1999) *Treating People with Depression: a practical guide for primary care*. Radcliffe Medical Press, Oxford.

WHO (1994) *Mental and Behavioural Disorders: ICD-10*. Churchill Livingstone, Edinburgh.

WHO (1996) *Diagnostic and Management Guidelines for Mental Disorders in Primary Care: ICD-10, Chapter V. Primary Care Version*. World Health Organisation/Hogrefe & Huber Publishers, Göttingen.

Van der Kolk B, Boyd H, Krystal J and Greenberg M (1984) Post-traumatic stress disorder as a biologically based disorder: implications of the animal model of inescapable shock. In: B Van der Kolk (ed.) *Post-Traumatic Stress Disorder: psychological and biological sequelae*. American Psychiatric Press, Washington, DC.

Appendix I:
Useful resources

Self-help books

Breton S (1996) *Don't Panic: a guide to overcoming panic attacks*. Macdonald Optima.

Lewis D (1997) *Fight Your Phobia and Win*. Sheldon Publishing.

MacFarlane M (1995) *The Panic Attack, Anxiety and Phobia Solutions Handbook*. United Research Publishers.

Marks I (1978) *Living with Fear*. McGraw-Hill.

Muir A (1993) *Step by Step: self-help for panic, anxiety and phobias*. Action on Phobias Association, Scotland.

Rachman S and de Silva P (1996) *Panic disorder: the facts*. Oxford University Press.

Sheehan D (1990) *The Anxiety Disease*. Bantam Books.

Stern R (1995) *Mastering Phobias: cases, causes and cures*. Penguin.

Help is at Hand Leaflets – written for the general public and produced by **The Royal College of Psychiatrists** (17 Belgrave Square, London SW1X 8PG). Leaflets entitled: *Social Phobias; Are You Sleeping Well? Alcohol and Depression; Depression in the Elderly; Depression in the Workplace; Postnatal Depression; Anxiety and Phobias; Bereavement; Depression; Manic Depression; Memory Disorders; Schizophrenia*. (Send a stamped addressed envelope: 20p for 1–3 copies, 64p for a sample set.)

Support groups, help lines and organisations

Emergencies:

The Samaritans
10 The Grove
Slough SL1 1QP
Tel: (admin) 01753 532713
National help-line 0345 909090

A national organisation offering support to those in distress who feel suicidal or despairing and need someone to talk to. The phone lines are open 24 hours a day, every day of the year. The number of your local branch can be found in the telephone directory or ask the operator.

Support groups and organisations

The National Phobic Society
407 Wilbraham Road
Chorlton
Manchester M21 0UT
Tel: 0161 881 1937

A network of branches where problems can be discussed. Also covers depression and obsessional problems. Provides printed information.

Triumph Over Phobia (TOP UK)
Flat One
4 Marlborough Buildings
Bath BA1 2LX
Tel: 01225 314129

Provides information and addresses of local self-help groups which use a structured approach to helping people overcome phobias.

Phobic Action Line
Mid Staffs Mind
Swiftbrook
Corporation Street
Stafford ST16 3LY
Help-line: 01785 211 144

No Panic
93 Brands Farm Way
Randlay, Telford
Shropshire TF3 2JQ
Help-line: 01952 590 545

Relaxation for Living
'Foxhills'
30 Victoria Avenue
Shanklin
Isle of Wight
PO37 6LS
Tel: 01983 868 166

Alternative address:
168–170 Oatlands Drive
Weybridge
Surrey KT13 9ET
Tel: 01932 831 000

Healthwise telephone service: (Freephone) 0800 665544
Free national help-line providing information and advice on any aspect
of health.

Smokers' QUITLINE: (Freephone) 0800 002200
Free national help-line providing help and advice for people wanting to
stop smoking. Provides telephone counselling and advice, sends free
information packs and refers to local Stop Smoking groups.

Alcoholics Anonymous
PO Box 1
Stonebow House
Stonebow
York YO1 7NJ
Tel: 01904 644 026
National help-line: 0171 833 0022

Drinkline – National help-line: 0800 917 8282
Mon–Fri 9 a.m.– 11 p.m.
Sat–Sun 6 p.m.–11 p.m.
Confidential alcohol counselling and information service.

Narcotics Anonymous – National help-line: 0171 730 0009
For advice, information and counselling on drug addiction.

Council for Involuntary Tranquiliser Addiction (CITA) – Help-line: 0151 949 0102

National Debtline – National help-line: 0645 500 511

CRUSE, bereavement care – National help-line: 0181 332 7227
Help-line for bereaved people and those caring for the bereaved. Can put you in contact with local counselling offices.

Women's Aid – National help-line: 0345 023 468
Help-line for women suffering from domestic violence.

RELATE (formerly Marriage Guidance Council)
Herbert Gray College
Little Church Street
Rugby
Warwickshire CV21 3AP
Tel: 01788 573 241

For access to a network of local counselling and advice centres.

Appendix 2
Self-monitoring sheets

Guidelines for 'normal behaviour' for those with obsessive-compulsive problems in washing and checking

Washing

1 Do not exceed one 10-minute shower daily

2 Do not exceed five hand-washings per day, 30 seconds each

3 Restrict hand-washing to when hands are visibly dirty or sticky

4 Continue to expose yourself deliberately on a weekly basis to objects or situations that used to disturb you

5 If objects or situations are still somewhat disturbing, expose yourself twice weekly to them

6 Do not avoid situations that cause discomfort. If you detect a tendency to avoid a situation, confront it deliberately at least twice a week

Checking

1 Do not check more than once any objects or situations that used to trigger an urge to check

2 Do not check even once in situations that your therapist has advised you do not require checking

3 Do not avoid situations that trigger an urge to check. If you detect a tendency to avoid, confront these situations deliberately twice a week and exercise control by not checking

4 Do not assign responsibility for checking to friends or family members in order to avoid checking

Self-help sheets for people with obsessive-compulsive problems.

Dealing with difficult behaviours/rituals:

- don't avoid, but approach difficult experiences
- remember, the best way to overcome your fear of something is to face it
- do daily relaxation – it will keep your anxiety levels down and your thoughts calm
- do relaxation before a difficult task
- organise your tasks and goals – give yourself plenty of time to do them
- choosing goals :
  - make them realistic and achievable
  - make goals and steps to them specific; what? where? when? with whom?
  - break up the goal into small steps
  - give yourself a time scale
- use recording sheets to plan and monitor your tasks
- try breathing exercises if you are in the middle of a task and it's getting the better of you
- reward yourself after achieving your task, look at the positive points even if it wasn't completed. Tell someone else about your achievement.

Dealing with distressing thoughts:

- let the thought drift through your mind when it comes out of the blue (i.e. when you're not doing a specific task)
- use distraction – switch to a pre-arranged thought pattern, e.g. imagine yourself eating your favourite meal
- use thought stopping – block the thought, say stop!, no! to yourself
- during tasks, use coping thoughts and rational answers:
- coping thoughts – one step at a time
  – just think about what you have to do
  – I'll just slow down until I feel better
  – the fear will pass, I know it doesn't last long
  – I've done this before, so I can do it again
  – I know it's never as bad as I think it will be
  – I'll have a go anyway, just give it a try
  – if I stick at this, I know next time will be easier
- rational answers come from a logical assessment of the situation
  – what evidence have I got to support these thoughts?
  – these thoughts are 'old' thoughts, they belong in the past
- tell yourself that each time you manage something, that's one more piece of evidence that you **can** do it without a disaster happening

Date: _____

Target: _____
_____
_____

Time: _____

Alone or accompanied: _____

If accompanied, by whom: _____

Anxiety (0–100)   Before: _____

                        During (highest): _____

                        After: _____

Any panics: _____

Comments: _____
_____
_____
_____

Ideas for next target: _____
_____
_____

Exposure practice chart.

© Wilkinson, Moore and Moore

Date:

Description of task:

For each stage listed, give your rating by circling the cross underneath the number which best describes *how you feel at the time*.
Do the rating *in the situation itself*, NOT later when you think back.

SITUATION	I don't feel at all uncomfortable										I feel the most uncomfortable I have ever felt
	0	10	20	30	40	50	60	70	80	90	100
_____	X	X	X	X	X	X	X	X	X	X	X
_____	X	X	X	X	X	X	X	X	X	X	X
_____	X	X	X	X	X	X	X	X	X	X	X
_____	X	X	X	X	X	X	X	X	X	X	X
_____	X	X	X	X	X	X	X	X	X	X	X
_____	X	X	X	X	X	X	X	X	X	X	X
_____	X	X	X	X	X	X	X	X	X	X	X
____ MINUTES LATER	X	X	X	X	X	X	X	X	X	X	X

Recording sheet for a behavioural test/experiment.

Situation	What I predict will happen	Negative thoughts about the situation	What actually happened	Change in thoughts afterwards

Monitoring changes in thoughts in response to exposure.

Rating scale
(0–100)

_____

1 _____ _____

2 _____ _____

3 _____ _____

4 _____ _____

5 _____ _____

6 _____ _____

7 _____ _____

8 _____ _____

9 _____ _____

10 _____ _____

Ideas to help you construct this hierarchy:

- looking at pictures of the stimulus, or watching films
- think of real-life situations
- watching someone else do it first
- doing things first with someone, then alone
- think of the things that make each task easier or harder – distance from the object, having particular people around, being in new or unfamiliar places

Hierarchy/fear ladder.

Thoughts Diary (A–B–C chart)

Date and time	Situation What were you doing? Anyone else there?	Emotions What did you feel? Rate 0–10	Thoughts Use exact words, How much did you believe them? Rate 0–10	Rational response What are your answers to the 'NATs'? How much do you believe them? Rate 0–10

Thoughts diary.

Balance sheet for thoughts

My thought: _____

EVIDENCE IN FAVOUR OF MY THOUGHT Note past situations where this thought was true	EVIDENCE AGAINST MY THOUGHTS Be alert for situations which disprove your negative thought

Thoughts balance sheet.

Patient's individualised sheet to prevent relapse

My setback sheet (or what to do if things slip back)
1 Don't shy away from doing things that are difficult. Do them quickly, before you have time to worry again
2 Remember how many times you had to visit the post office before you felt OK. Now even the shops in town are OK
3 Do the relaxation exercises properly once a month as a reminder. (NB Write this in diary so it doesn't get forgotten)
4 Don't get bogged down in the horror of it all: it's more encouraging to think about the progress I have made before, and what to do next. Write down the steps involved
5 Look back at old record sheets. They show which order I did things before, and how much practice I had to do before it got easier
6 Go into the supermarket alone sometimes. Don't always go with the family, even if it's more convenient to do so
7 Plan to go to all the school concerts next term
8 Breathe slowly when you feel bad
9 Watch out for thinking the worst will happen. It hasn't happened yet!

If things get difficult again:

- Remember setbacks happen to everyone. You can't get through life without having some bad times

- Work out how to practise in steps. Write the steps down, and make sure you tackle them one by one. Write down how you felt each time

- Practise every day. There's no need to run before you can walk

- Don't bottle it up. Talk to the family about what's happening

Panic diary

Date and time	Situation	Rate severity (0–100)	Bodily sensations	Negative interpretation (rate belief 0–100)	Rational response (rerate belief 0–100)

Panic diary.

Patient's plan of action for setbacks

What to do if my panic returns

- If I notice that I am becoming increasingly sensitive to my heartbeat and starting to have frightening thoughts and images:
  - restart my daily recordings, trying to find out what may be triggering the thoughts
  - once I know the triggers, set down the evidence for and against at least two alternative explanations and make plans to test these out
- If I find myself starting to avoid situations for reasons of fear, that is the surest sign that I need to:
  - enter those situations repeatedly and
  - remain there for increasing periods until the panic symptoms disappear

Holmes and Rahe's hassles scale

Life events and stress

Life event	Stress rating
Death of a spouse	100
Divorce or marital separation	73
Jail term	63
Death of close family member	63
Personal injury or illness	53
Marriage	50
Loss of job	47
Moving house	45
Marital reconciliation	45
Retirement	45
Serious illness of family member	44
Pregnancy	40
Sexual difficulties	39
Birth of a new child	39
Change of job	39
Financial problems	38
Death of a close friend	37
Increase in family disharmony	35
High mortgage	31
Legal action over debt	30
Change in work responsibilities	29
Children leaving home	29
Trouble with in-laws	29
Outstanding personal achievement	28
Spouse begins or stops work	26
Children beginning or ending school	26
Change in living conditions	25
Revision of personal habits	24
Trouble with boss	23
Change in work hours or conditions	20
Change in children's school	20
Change in recreation or leisure pursuits	19
Change in church activities	19
Change in social activities	18
Small mortgage or loan	17
Change in sleeping habits	16
Change in contact with family	15
Change in eating habits	15
Holidays	13
Christmas	12
Minor violations of the law	11

Scoring:

Below 60	– A life unusually free of stress
60–80	– Normal amount of stress
80–100	– Stress in life rather high
100+	– Under serious stress at home, work or both

This exercise is not meant to be taken too seriously – just to give an idea of the various sources of stress in our modern lives.

Date and time	Situation and general feeling	Distressing thoughts	Anxiety level 0–100	Checking/rituals – actions or thoughts	How long did it last? How many times?	Did you manage to stop? How?	Who else involved in checking?

Monitoring sheet for checking compulsions.

© Wilkinson, Moore and Moore

Patient's 'setback sheet'

- Take things in steps, don't take on something I am not ready to handle
- Tasks that you decide to do should be handled in stages, don't worry if some are not mastered, you will have some 'off days'. Don't give up because one time didn't work out right
- After doing tasks, however distressing, the thing to remember is that anxiety will come down
- Use relaxation techniques to help here
- All thoughts, however distressing, should be taken hold of and analysed, retraining my mind
- Remember the things that help:
  - letting thoughts and anxieties float over you, let them flow straight through your mind
  - answering worrying thoughts so that a crazy, mixed-up thought becomes a more level-headed, reasonable thought, more like reality than fantasy
  - taking control of situations like counting
- Allow myself to feel feelings. It is not wrong to feel or think anything
- Talk to people; don't bottle up feelings and anxieties
- When thoughts come, if you can think them through without acting on them by checking, half the battle's won

Index